The
Warfighter
Nutrition
Guide

Human Performance Resource Center

Consortium for Health and Military Performance (CHAMP)

Uniformed Services University of the Health Sciences (USUHS)

1 The Warrior Athlete

WF
Olympic Athletes
Professional Athletes
Marines and Other Specialty Units
College Athletes
High School and Recreational Athletes
Rest of Population

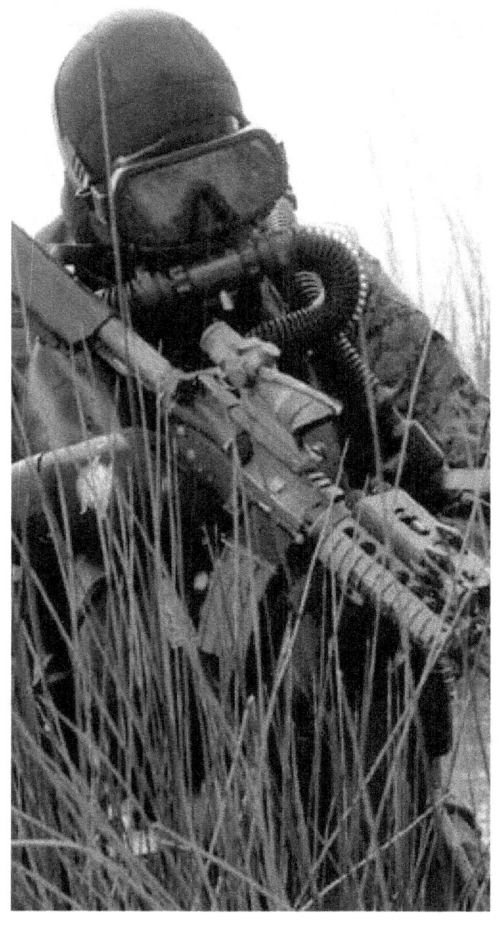

Nutrition for the Warfighter

The demands imposed by military service, training, and missions are unlike any athletic endeavor. Success requires the mustering of all strength and endurance—both physical and mental. Military service members, Warfighters (WF), are indeed "Warrior Athletes," the ultimate athlete, at the top of the athletic pyramid. One factor that will contribute to mission success and life-long health is good nutrition. It is well known that appropriate nutritional habits and interventions can enhance performance, and these successful approaches need to be known.

Warfighter	Professional/Olympic Athlete
Year-round training cycle.	Seasonal training.
Multiple skills.	One sport.
Volunteer.	Sponsored.
24/7 potential for deployment.	Well scheduled and orchestrated events.
Self-trained/Help yourself.	Full spectrum support.
Eat on the fly/Help yourself.	Sports nutritionist/Psychologists.
Military issue tents.	Pampered with 5-star hotels.
Covert ops.	Limelight and enthusiastic audience.
Life/Death.	Win/Lose.
Global impact.	Self-promotion/Local enthusiasm.
Unexpected is the norm.	Structured and controlled.
Private reflection and satisfaction.	Money, endorsements, Olympic gold, public approval, and appreciation.
Unit at risk.	Team effort.
Buddy-reliant.	Coach-directed goals.

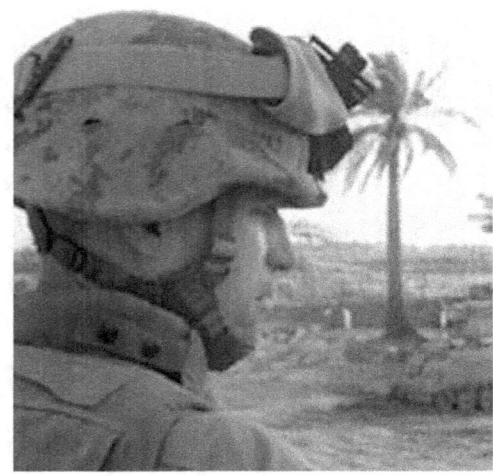

All service members are Warfighters, regardless of duties. This manual is intended to be a resource for all Warfighters and includes a variety of materials ranging from short summaries to detailed information, with worksheets, links, and important tips for nutrition at home and when deployed.

Looking Forward

This Nutrition Guide evolved into the final product after multiple conversations, discussions, and interactions with miltary, fitness, and nutrition experts. The Guide is dense, but each chapter starts with key information, and an executive summary provides a "shortened" version.

- Chapters 2 through 4 provide general background information about energy expenditure, source of energy, essential nutrients and nutrition concepts. These are the backbone of the guide.

- Chapters 5 through 8 will help you select a healthy diet: they contain menus for eating at home, menus for eating in ethnic and fast food restaurants, choosing healthy snacks, selecting appropriate military rations, and combining commercial-off-the-shelf products with military rations.

- Chapters 9 through 13 review important information on being a warrior athlete. Detailed information and websites that discuss dietary supplements, combat rations and products to be avoided are also provided.

- Chapters 14 and 15 explore nutritional strategies for various missions, how to optimize nutritional intake to combat challenging environmental and physiological conditions, and how to eat on the local economy when deployed.

- Chapter 16 discusses nutritional strategies to regain pre-deployment health and fitness after returning home from extended deployments.

- Chapters 17 and 18 provide information on how to be a warrior athlete for 20+ years and what the "high-mileage" warrior athlete should consider in order to maintain operational readiness and good health after years of physical abuse.

Future Success

Warfighters are a select group of warrior athletes who can benefit from nutritional guidance. Each command has specialized missions, with the duration of deployments ranging from 30 days to 12 months. Long missions in locations far from the central support hub pose very difficult nutritional challenges to Warfighters, and unfortunately, good solutions are not always possible. Despite differences across military commands, this guide has been designed to cover the spectrum of needs, so performance under the most rigorous conditions is optimized. The success of Warfighters require effective nutritional strategies to optimize performance during operations and preserve health during the golden years of retirement.

All service members are Warfighters. All Warfighters are "warrior athletes."

2 Balancing the Energy Tank

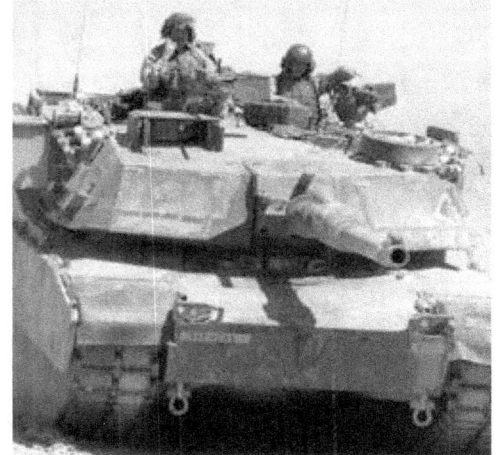

Key Points

- Balancing energy intake and expenditure can be difficult when activity levels are very high and also when activity levels are very low, such as during isolation.

- Typically, body weight remains constant when energy intake equals expenditure.

- To lose or gain one pound of weight, 3,500 calories must be expended or consumed.

- Calculating Resting Energy Expenditure (REE) and the intensity of daily activities gives an accurate estimate of how much energy a Warfighter might expend in one day.

- The Body Mass Index (BMI) is a clinical tool for assessing body fat composition and classifies individuals into underweight, normal, over-weight, and obese categories.

Energy balance is one very important aspect of nutrition. Knowing how much energy is going to be expended allows one to calculate how much fuel the "tank" requires to function and how much fuel to take on missions. Energy expenditure must be balanced by energy intake to maintain body weight or "energy balance." To determine how much fuel your tank needs, basic information about metabolic rate and activity level is needed. This chapter will address those issues.

Units of Energy

The unit most commonly used to describe energy intake and energy expenditure is the **calorie**. The terms **kilocalorie** (kcal) and **kilojoule** are also used when referring to energy intake and expenditure. For simplicity:

- 1 kcal = 1 calorie.

Throughout this book we will use the terms kcal and calorie interchangeably.

Sensitivity of Energy Balance

The energy balance equation can be "unbalanced" by changing energy intake, energy expenditure, or both. To gain or lose 1 pound, approximately 3,500 extra kcal must be consumed or expended. Believe it or not, the energy balance equation is very sensitive.

$$1 \text{ lb} = 3{,}500 \text{ kcal.}$$

Example 1:

- One 32 oz Gatorade® has 4 servings of 8 fl oz. If you consumed the whole bottle, you would drink 200 kcal (8 oz = 50 kcal).

- If you drank one 32 oz Gatorade® per day every day of the year without increasing your activity level, you would add 73,000 kcal (200 x 365 days/yr), which is 20.8 lbs in one year.

Example 2:

- Eating one PowerBar® Protein Plus per day would provide 258 kcal of energy.

- Eating one PowerBar® Protein Plus per day for an entire year without increasing your activity level, would add 94,170 kcal (258 x 365 days/yr), which is 26.9 lbs per year.

Example 3:

- Drinking one extra beer per day would provide an additional 145 kcal of energy.

- Drinking one beer per day for an entire year without increasing your activity level, would add 52,925 kcal (145 x 365 days/year), which is 15.1 lbs per year.

Components of Energy Expenditure

The three major contributors to energy expenditure are:

- Resting energy expenditure.
- Physical activity.
- Energy for digesting foods (TEF or thermic effect of food).

The first two are of interest here and will be discussed in detail.

Resting Energy Expenditure (REE):

The amount of energy required to maintain life.

Table 2–1. Determining Resting Energy Expenditure (REE) of Men From Body Weight (in pounds)

Age (yrs)	Equation to Derive REE (kcal/day)
18–30	6.95 x Weight + 679
31–60	5.27 x Weight + 879

Resting Energy Expenditure

Resting Energy Expenditure (REE) is the amount of energy required to maintain life—such as breathing, beating of the heart, maintaining body temperature, and other life processes. Measurements are made in the morning after waking with the body at complete rest. REE can be estimated by a formula to predict your daily energy requirements. The only information needed is your body weight in pounds.

Physical Activity Energy Expenditure

The amount of energy you expend during physical activity is different each day, depending on your training. Some days are very strenuous and involve running, swimming, calisthenics, cold water exposure, sleep deprivation, and carrying heavy loads. Some days you are in the classroom sitting a good portion of the day. Thus, determining your actual energy expended during activity is more difficult, but there are ways to estimate it. You would usually take your REE and multiply it by a number (or factor) based on your expected physical activity, as shown in Table 2–2. Multiplying your REE by this physical activity factor provides a rough estimate of your total energy/calorie needs.

Example:

You are 21, weigh 175 lbs, and activity is moderate.

REE = 6.95 x Weight + 679 = 6.95 x 175 + 679 = 1,895 kcal/day.

Total Energy Needs = 1,895 x 1.7 = 3,222 kcal/day.

Note: Formula for REE came from Table 2–1; 1.7 is the Activity Factor for "Moderate Activity."

How to Calculate Energy Expenditure

You will need a calculator to complete this exercise.

Over a 24-hour period, different amounts of energy will be expended in each activity you engage in, be it watching TV, eating, running in boots, humping, or listening to teammates. The objective of this activity is to increase awareness of the energy actually expended.

- Record your name and date on the Energy Expenditure Activity Form.

- List all the activities participated in over the last 12 hours and the

General Activity	**Activity Factor (x REE)**
Very Light: Seated and standing activities, driving, playing cards.	1.3
Light: Walking, carpentry, sailing, playing ping-pong or pool, golf.	1.6
Moderate: Carrying a load, jogging, light swimming, biking, calisthenics, scuba diving.	1.7
Heavy: Walking with a load uphill, rowing, digging, climbing, soccer, basketball, running, obstacle course.	2.1
Exceptional: Running/swimming races, cycling uphill, carrying very heavy loads, hard rowing.	2.4

Table 2–1. Physical Activity Factor for Various Levels of Activity

Activity	Time (minutes)	Energy Value (kcal/ minute)	Total Calories (kcal)
Name:		Date:	
Obstacle course	30	10	300
4-mile run, 8-min/mile pace	32	14	448
Calisthenics	30	8	240
Weight lifting	45	11	495
14-mile run in boots	140	12	1680
5-mile hike w/80 lb load	100	14	1400
Grand Total		4,563 kcal	

approximate length of time (in minutes) spent on each activity.

- Go through the alphabetical list of activities, and find the activity that most closely approximates the ones you listed on the form.

- Write down on the form the kcal/minute (not per hour!) value in the appropriate column (Energy Value).

- Multiply the energy value by the total time in minutes. For example, if you ran in boots for 25 minutes, then your energy expenditure for that activity would be 12 (energy value) x 25 (time) = 300 kcals.

Do this for five activities, or preferably all events in 12 hours. Then add up the numbers to get an actual energy expenditure estimate. How did you fare? Keep track of your weight if you are in doubt—it is the most accurate way to monitor energy balance.

Body Size and Body Mass Index

Body Mass Index, or BMI, is a measure commonly used to rapidly assess body composition and classify individuals as underweight, normal, overweight or obese. BMI is the ratio of (weight in kg)/(height in m)^2, or [(weight in lb) x 704.5]/(height in inches)^2. Reference standards have been developed for the United States population by race and gender, so that individuals at risk for obesity can be easily identified. However, the reference values for the U.S. population do not always apply to special populations, such as Warfighters. As a result, unique populations often develop their own standards and references based on individuals within that population. A reference range based on a survey of over 800 SEAL Warfighters was developed. The average BMI was 25, and the average body fat was 13%.

BMI is a screening tool, and you can use it to keep track of changes in your body composition. If your BMI is high, have your body fat checked, and if your body fat is more than 20%, you should take action to lower your weight.

3 Fueling the Human Weapon

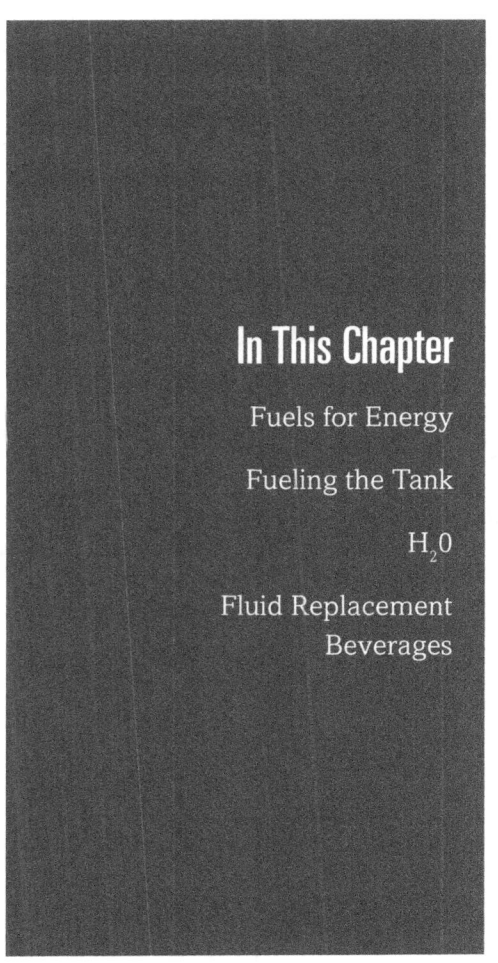

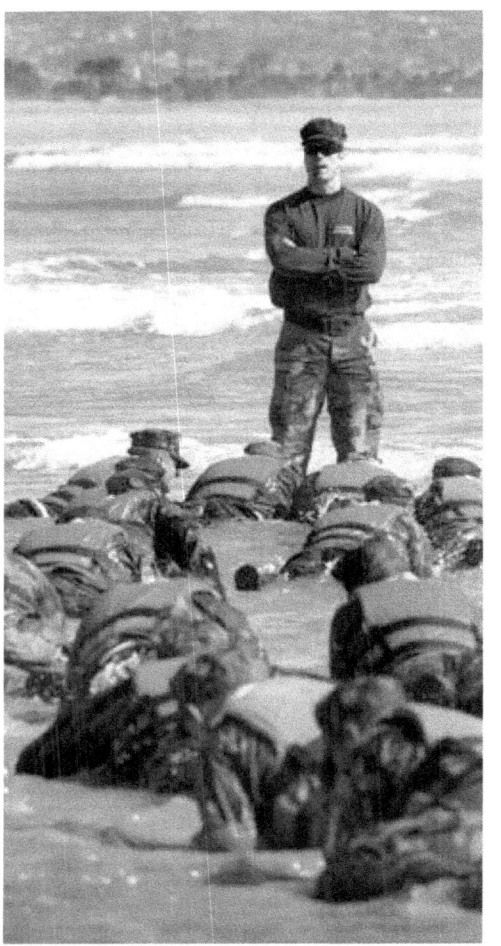

Key Points

- Carbohydrates (CHO) are the vital fuel for endurance and resistance activities, competitive athletic events, mental agility, and healthy living.

- Fats, the primary form of stored energy, are essential, but should be eaten in moderation.

- Proteins are essential for building and repairing body tissues; however, excess protein is converted to fat.

- Restore fluid balance by taking in enough liquids to replenish weight (pounds) lost plus an additional 25%.

- Performance decrements begin when only 2% of body weight has been lost.

"You Are What You Eat." Although this statement has not been proven, it is known that the foods eaten make a difference in performance, longevity, and quality of life. A car engine typically uses only one source of fuel, but the body can use carbohydrate, fat, protein, and alcohol. To a certain extent, the source of fuel is dictated by availability. In other words, the body tends to use whatever it has. The macronutrients, or energy-providing nutrients, are important in this respect. Without energy the body would starve, and performance would be greatly reduced. The three main sources of energy are:

- Carbohydrate.

- Fat.

- Protein.

These fuels are called "macronutrients' because they are eaten in large quantities unlike the micronutrients to be discussed later. This chapter will provide basic information about macronutrients and alcohol, which may be a dominant source of energy among Warfighters. In addition, information relating to portion size and hydration will be provided.

8

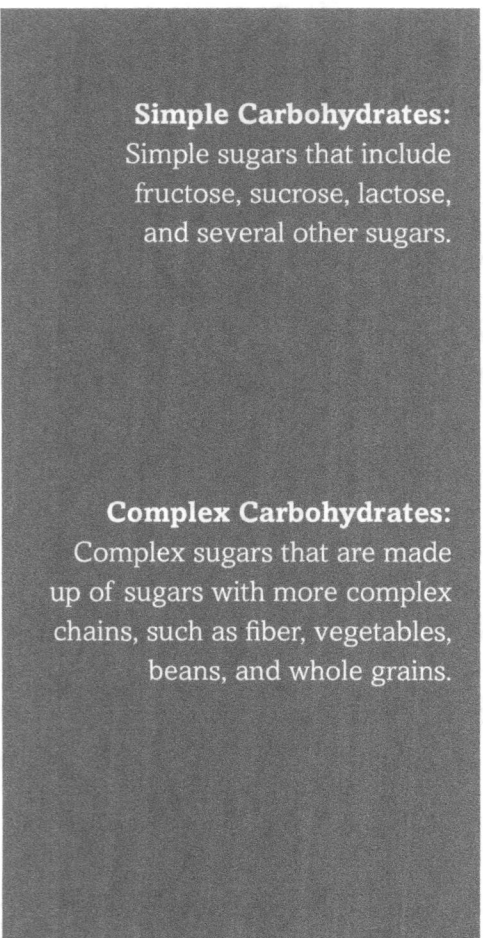

Simple Carbohydrates:
Simple sugars that include fructose, sucrose, lactose, and several other sugars.

Complex Carbohydrates:
Complex sugars that are made up of sugars with more complex chains, such as fiber, vegetables, beans, and whole grains.

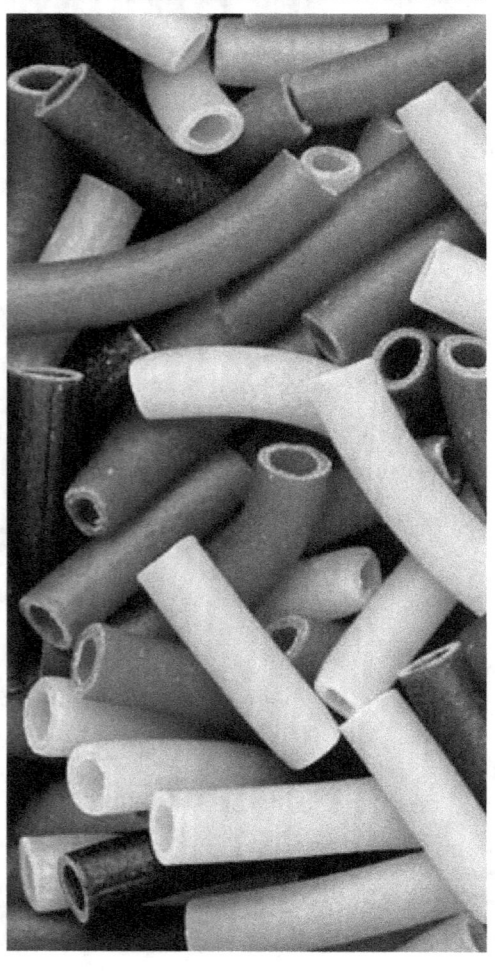

Fuels for Energy

Carbohydrates

Carbohydrates, or CHO, are the preferred foods for endurance and resistance training, competitive athletic events, mental agility, and healthy living. CHO foods are the preferred energy source for all athletes and for Warfighters. CHO should not be restricted. In the past, CHO have been considered "off-limits" and many Warfighters have blamed weight gain on CHO. In addition, many fad diets promote protein and fat at the expense of CHO, but as a vital energy source, and restriction can degrade performance. Chapters 5, 9 and 10 discuss the amount of CHO to eat with respect to nutrient timing and type of training.

Definition, Composition, and Classification

Carbohydrates exist in many forms, but the two major types of CHO are labelled simple and complex.

- Simple CHO include table sugar, honey, fruit sugars, milk sugar, brown sugar, corn syrup, maple syrup, corn sweeteners, high-fructose corn syrup, and molasses.

- Complex CHO include grains, fruits, seeds, potatoes, pasta, seaweed, algae, peas and beans, and all other vegetables.

- Complex CHO, starches and fibers, come from plant materials. The body digests starches, but it does not digest dietary fiber. Fiber is discussed in Chapter 18.

Functions of Carbohydrate in the Body

CHO are used in the body mainly as:

- Fuel for muscles, brain, heart, and other organs in the form of glucose; the brain requires 130 grams/day from glucose.

- Building blocks to make chemicals needed by the body.

- Chemical cement for joints and other structures in your body.

- Glycogen is the only CHO stored in humans.

Glycogen, stored in liver and skeletal muscle, is limited to about 500 grams and is depleted by three to four hours of heavy exercise; a 24-hour fast will use up liver glycogen stores.

Carbohydrate in the Diet

Some people are phobic about eating CHO and believe that foods high in CHO are unhealthy and lead to weight gain. Fear **not**. That notion comes from muscle-building myths and low CHO diet fads that lack scientific evidence. No one has ever been able to show that performance suffers from consuming potatoes, rice and bread. To the contrary, performance is enhanced by such foods. Rather, high-fat toppings (butter on bread, sour cream on potatoes, cream cheese on bagels, cream sauces on macaroni) may contribute to the notion that CHO are bad. Also, CHO that are highly processed with high fructose corn syrup and other highly processed sugars, are less healthy than whole food products, such as baked potatoes, brown rice, whole wheat pasta, and wheat bread. CHO-rich foods from around the world are shown below.

Table 3–1. Carbohydrate Sources in Selected Countries	
Country	**Carbohydrates in food***
Mexico	Corn tortillas, beans.
Brazil	Black beans, rice.
India	Chick peas (garbanzo beans), lentils, rice, whole grain unleavened breads.
Japan	Rice, tofu, vegetables.
Middle East	Hummus (chick peas), tahini (sesame seeds).
United States	Bread, potatoes, noodles, macaroni.

*When combined, these CHO are also a good source of protein.

Energy From Carbohydrate

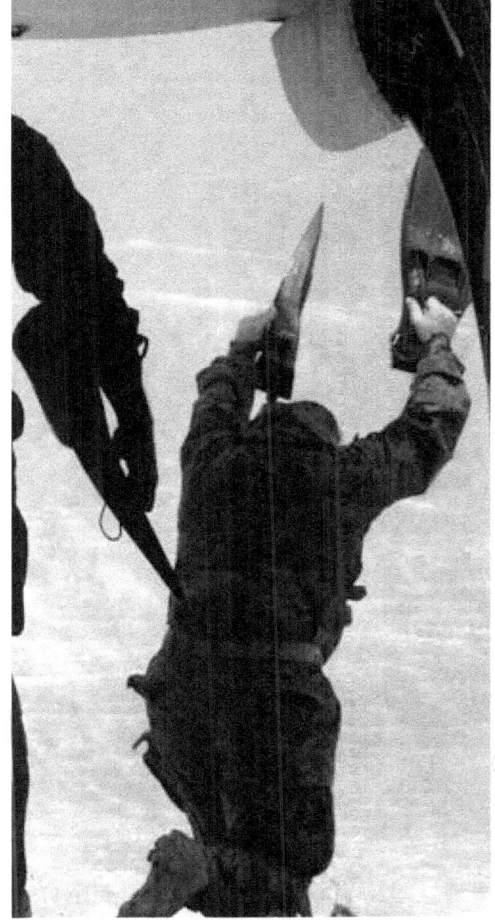

One gram of Carbohydrate = 4 kcal.

Fat

Fat is a vital part of the diet as it adds taste to foods and satisfies hunger. However, not all fats are created equal. By understanding the different types of dietary fat, how it works in the body, and using guidelines for daily

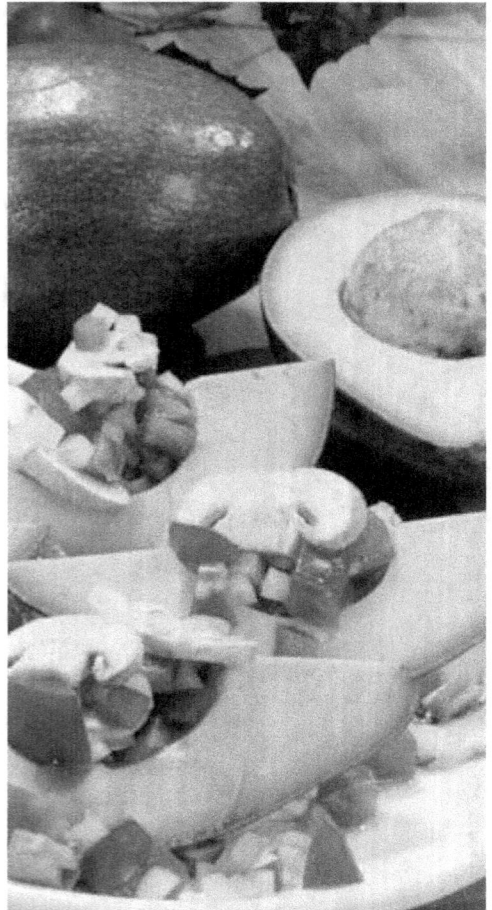

fat consumption, excess fat can be eliminated from your diet and you can eat for better health.

Definition, Composition, and Classification

Fat (technically fatty acids) is an essential nutrient and is usually classified according to its chemical form.

Type	Description	Examples
Saturated Fats	Solid at room temperature.	Whole milk, cream, ice cream, whole-milk cheeses, butter, lard, meat, palm kernel, coconut oils, and cocoa butter.
Polyunsaturated Fats	Liquid at room temperature.	Safflower, sesame, soy, corn and sunflower-seed oils, nuts, seeds, and fish.
Monounsaturated Fats	Liquid at room temperature but may solidify in the refrigerator.	Olive oil, canola and peanut oil, peanut butter, cashews, almonds, and avocados.
Trans Fats or "Partially Hydrogenated" Fats	Man-made from saturated fats.	Cookies, crackers, and other commercial baked goods, French fries, donuts, fried onion rings and other commercial fried foods.

Functions of Fat in the Body

Fat serves a number of critical functions:

- Major form of stored energy: provides energy during exercise, in cold environments, and during starvation.

- Insulates the body.

- Helps transport other nutrients to places in the body.

- Protects organs.

- Serves a structural role in cells.

How Much Fat Should We Eat?

All the different types of fats are desirable, but **too** much fat is the primary dietary problem in our country. A high intake of fat is associated with many diseases, including:

- Heart disease.

- Obesity.

- Many forms of cancer.

- Diabetes.

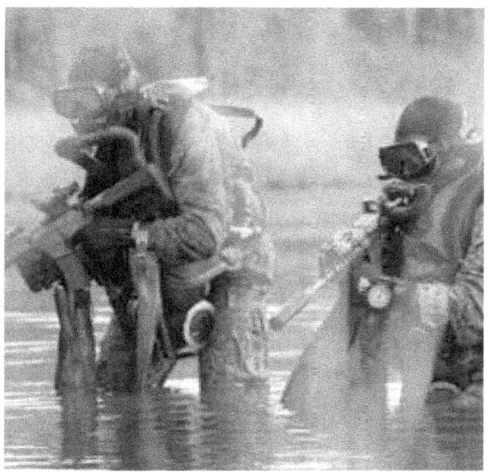

The average American consumes 33% of daily calories as fat (52% carbohydrate and 15% protein). Total fat intake (saturated, trans, monounsaturated, polyunsaturated) should be adjusted to fit total caloric needs. It is recommended that no more than 35% of total calories come from fat. Saturated fat intake should not exceed 10% and the balance should come from mono- and poly-unsaturated fats. Trans fat intake should be less than 1% of total calories each day.

Energy From Fat

One gram of FAT = 9 kcal.

Fat provides more than twice the
energy supplied by CHO and protein.

Determining Your Daily Fat Allowance

Everyone talks about grams of fat, but what does that mean on a practical level? How does one translate "grams" of fat to percent fat and how many grams of fat should be consumed each day? Again, no more than 35% of calories should come from fat, so with that in mind, the example below will show you how to determine your daily fat allowance.

Example: Determining Fat Allowance

If estimated energy need (EEN)= 3,222 calories

Step 1. Multiply EEN by 0.35 to get calories from fat
3,222 x 0.35 = 1,128 fat calories

Step 2. Divide fat calories by 9 to get grams of fat.
1,128/9 = 125 grams of Fat per day

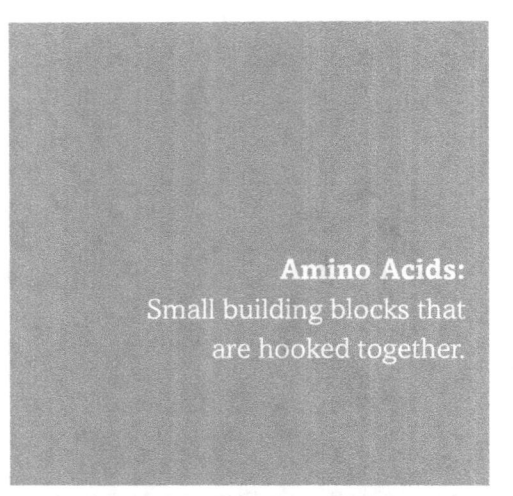

Amino Acids: Small building blocks that are hooked together.

Table 3–2. How Many Grams of Protein Do I Need?	
Activity Level	**Protein Range (grams/lb)**
Low to Moderate	0.4–0.5
Endurance Training	0.6–0.8
Strength/Weight Training	0.6–0.8

Over 1.6 grams of protein/pound body weight may compromise muscle growth.

Example: Suppose a Warfighter weighs 175 pounds and is training for a mission that requires both endurance and strength.

Protein needs = 0.6 x 175 lb = 105 grams

Protein needs = 0.9 x 175 lb = 140 grams

Protein needs = 105–140 g/day.

Where Did The Numbers Come From?

Estimated Energy Need or EEN was given to you in the example. You should know your EEN from the preceding chapter.

- 0.35 in Step 1 is for calculating 35% of calories from fat.
- 9 in Step 2 represents the number of calories in one gram of fat.
- 125 is the maximum number of grams of fat that should be eaten to ensure the diet provides no more than 35% of calories from fat.

An excel worksheet is provided to determine the amount of calories from you should get from the fat in your food.

Protein

Protein seems to be the preferred food among Warfighters to consume, based on the number of protein drinks and sports bars used in place of "real food." Also, people like to eat high protein foods because they think protein makes them grow "big and strong." Are they correct? Let's take a look at protein and what it really does.

Definition and Composition

CHO and fat consist of carbon, oxygen, and hydrogen; protein consists of these atoms, plus nitrogen, which is essential for life. Proteins are made up of amino acids—small building blocks hooked together in various orders. Although over 20 different amino acids are part of our body, only 10 are "essential amino acids" (EAA) because our body cannot make them; they must be obtained from protein in the diet. Failure to obtain enough of the 10 EAA, in the right balance, may result in degradation of other proteins, such as muscle, to obtain the one EAA that is needed. Unlike fats and starch, the human body does not store excess amino acids for later use—the amino acids must be obtained from the food every day.

The 10 EAA, in alphabetical order, are arginine (required for the young, but not for adults), histidine, isoleucine, leucine, lysine, methionine, phenylalanine, threonine, tryptophan, and valine.

Functions of Protein in the Body

Proteins vary in size, depending on how many amino acids are linked together, and each one performs different functions in the body. Although they can provide energy, protein is **not** a main source of energy, like carbohydrates and fat. Some functions of protein are:

- Muscle contraction.
- Formation of muscle, hair, nails, skin, and other tissues.
- Direct energy production.

- Repair of injuries.

- Transport fats, vitamins and minerals around the body.

- Structural roles for every part of the body.

How Much Protein Should I Eat?

Protein needs are determined by age, body weight, and activity level. Many athletes believe that if they eat more protein, their muscles will increase in size, but this is not true. Excess calories from protein can be converted to and stored as fat. Additionally, large quantities of protein strain the liver and the kidneys.

Energy from Protein

One gram of protein supplies 4 kcal.

Table 3–3. Summary of Macronutrients / Water

1 gram of...	=	kcal/g
Carbohydrate	=	4
Fat	=	9
Protein	=	4
Alcohol	=	7
Water	=	0

Alcohol

Alcoholic beverages (beer, wine, or liquor) are a potent source of energy, but they are not good sources of energy for physical activity or exercise. Obviously, alcohol is not essential, unlike CHO, protein and fat. Also, most people tend to eat junk food when they are drinking. If trying to keep in shape, it is a good idea to minimize the amount of alcohol consumed; it contains little in the way of other nutrients, so replacing a meal with alcohol is not a good idea.

One 12 oz beer is about 150 kcal and one 12 oz "lite" beer is approximately 110 kcal. Wine provides about 90 kcal for every 5 oz, and liquor contains 90 kcal for every 1.5 oz If the liquor is prepared with a carbonated drink, the energy intake will increase by at least 75 more kcal.

Energy from Alcohol

One gram of alcohol supplies 7 kcal.

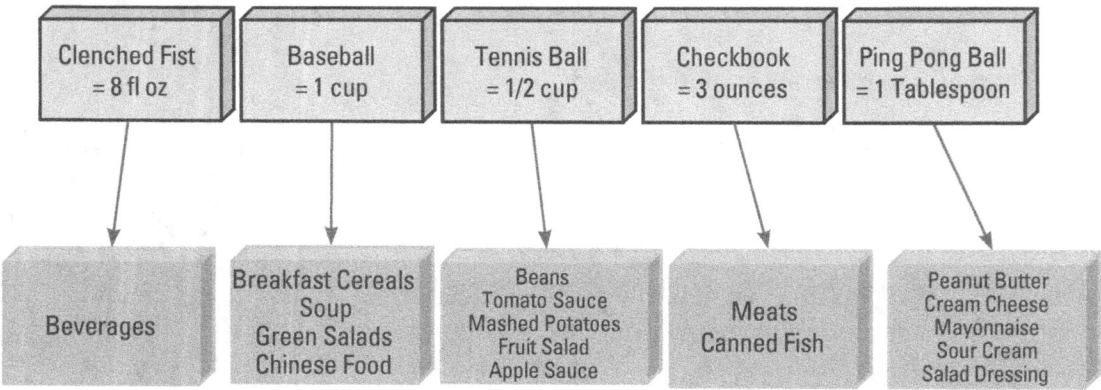

Clenched Fist = 8 fl oz	Baseball = 1 cup	Tennis Ball = 1/2 cup	Checkbook = 3 ounces	Ping Pong Ball = 1 Tablespoon
Beverages	Breakfast Cereals Soup Green Salads Chinese Food	Beans Tomato Sauce Mashed Potatoes Fruit Salad Apple Sauce	Meats Canned Fish	Peanut Butter Cream Cheese Mayonnaise Sour Cream Salad Dressing

Fueling the Tank

The term "serving" describes the recommended amount of food that should be eaten from each food group. Packaged foods list the number of servings on the Nutrition Facts panel and a serving describes the amount of food recommended in the Food Guide Pyramid and the Dietary Guidelines for Americans. A "portion" is the amount of a specific food chosen to be eaten or served for breakfast, lunch, dinner, or snack. Portions can be bigger or smaller than the recommended food servings. Over the past 20 years, portions have increased substantially, and this has resulted in many people eating more than they should. Larger portions have also contributed to the high incidence of obesity. The next page provides a summary of standard serving sizes, but a Serving Size Card can be downloaded, cut out, and laminated for long time use to help you recall what standard food servings look like.

H_2O

Water is an essential nutrient and the most abundant component of the human body. Approximately 50–70% of your total body weight is water. Since lean body/muscle mass requires more water than fat, the leaner one is, the more body water there is. Water must be consumed regularly to ensure normal functioning of the body.

Distribution and Functions of Water

Water is found inside and outside cells, but most water is inside cells, especially muscle cells. Water in the body serves many important roles, including:

- Participates in digestion and absorption of nutrients.
- Participates in excretion of wastes.
- Maintains blood circulation in the body.
- Maintains body temperature.

Table 3–4. Body Weight Losses and Dehydration	
Starting Weight (lbs)	2.5% Weight Change (lbs)
150	146
170	166
190	185

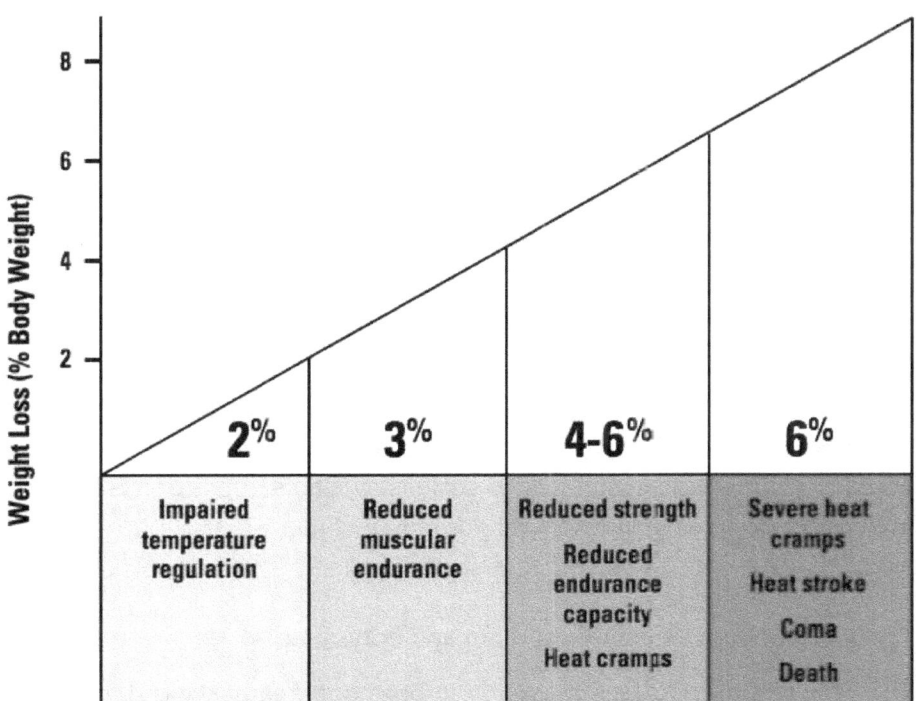

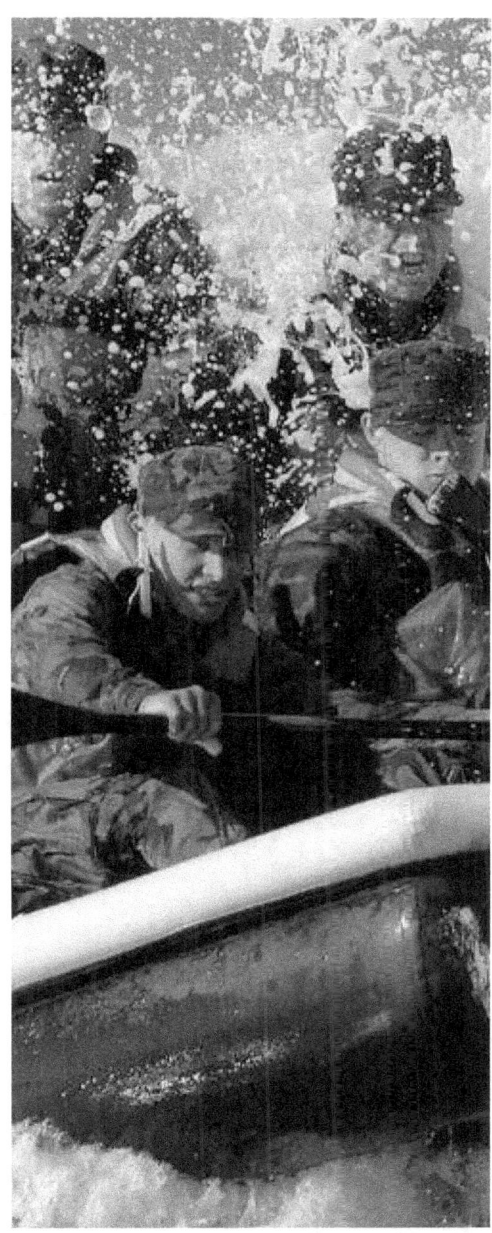

A loss of 2.5% of your body weight will result in performance decrements: decision-making and concentration will be impaired and 35% of physical performance potential can be lost.

Being well hydrated during operations is absolutely critical, since adequate fluids will help compensate for blood losses if wounded. For these reasons, fluid balance is essential to a Warfighter's performance. Below are signs and symptoms that might be experienced when weight is lost from dehydration.

- Thirsty.

- Dry mouth.

- Urine output reduced.

- Reduced physical performance.

- Headache and feeling ill.

- Difficulty concentrating.

- Sleepiness.

Maintaining Water Balance

Water balance is determined by water/fluid output and input. In order to maintain performance, it is critical that a fluid deficit or dehydration does not occur. With dehydration, water output exceeds input and balance becomes negative. A sedentary man typically will expel body water at a rate of 1–3.2 quarts (1–3 liters or 32–102 oz) a day from the following:

Table 3–5. Using Weight Loss to Estimate Fluids Replacement

Weight Lost (lbs)	Fluid to be Replaced (oz/cups)
1	20–24 (2.5–3 cups)
2	40 to 48 (5–6 cups)
4	80–96 (10–12 cups)
8	160–192 (20–24 cups)

The easiest way to restore fluid balance is by drinking fluids that contain sodium. This is **very** important to remember.

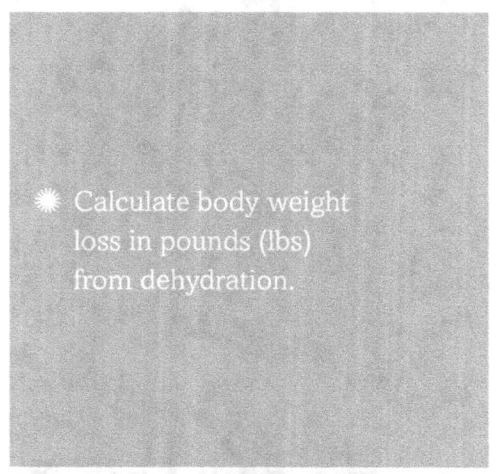

❋ Calculate body weight loss in pounds (lbs) from dehydration.

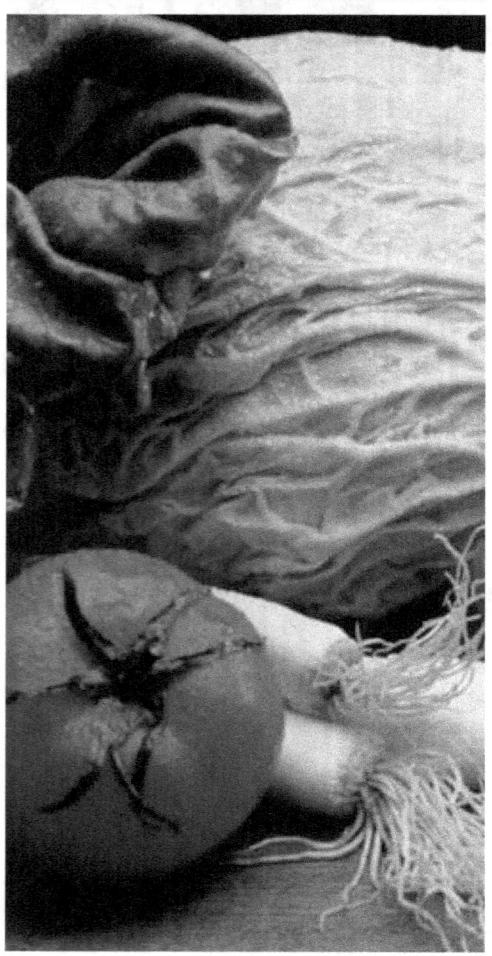

- Urine and stools.

- Breathing.

- Sweating.

When activity levels are low, most fluids are lost through the urine. However, when activity levels and/or the outdoor temperature are high, most fluid is lost by sweating. Up to 2.1 quarts (2 liters or 66 oz) per hour can be lost through sweating, depending on the outside temperatures and intensity of the activity.

All fluids lost must be added back each day by drinking 125–150% of the weight lost to restore fluid balance. This can be measured by weighing yourself as often as possible. If no scale is available, monitor the color of your urine. Sources of fluid for rehydrating include:

- Water in food.

- Sports drinks that contain sodium and potassium.

Sweat output increases markedly in both hot weather and during prolonged exercise—the amounts will be even greater if exercise is performed in the heat.

Eating foods high in water and drinking fluids will help restore water balance. The fresh foods listed in Table 3–6 are over 90% water. Beware of drinking too much plain water (hyper hydrating). It is also important to consume some sodium, which helps restore hydration status better than water taken alone. Taking in salt will also help prevent levels of sodium in the blood from getting too low (hyponatremia), which can be dangerous. Hyponatremia is a huge operational problem. It is caused by excessive intake of plain water during prolonged exercise. Salty foods can be ingested before or with other fluids (including sports drinks) to provide sodium, promote fluid retention, and stimulate fluid intake.

Table 3–6. Fresh Foods Containing Mainly Water			
Bean Sprouts	Broccoli	Cabbage	Carrots
Cauliflower	Celery	Cucumbers	Eggplant
Lettuce	Peaches	Spinach	Squash
Strawberries	Tomatoes	Watercress	Watermelon

What Conditions Will Increase Water Losses?

The primary ways in which you may become dehydrated, or in need of additional body fluids, are by:

- Exercising for over 60 minutes.

- Working in a hot environment—wet or dry.

- Working in a cold environment—wet or dry.

- Going to high altitudes.

- Drinking too much alcohol or caffeine.

- Exercising in the heat, cold, or at altitude.

- Exercising with a hangover.

☐	1
☐	2
☐	3
☐	4
☐	5
☐	6
☐	7
☐	8
☐	9

Several points about fluids should be considered:

- Do not rely on thirst as a good indicator of fluid needs; body weight losses are better.

- Before any exercise or simulated-mission, fluids should be ingested in anticipation of losing fluid (12–20 oz of cool water before exercise).

- Before starting, urine should be clear or between 1–3 on the chart (unless taking B vitamin supplements)—this is a sign of adequate hydration. The more dehydrated, the darker (and smellier) urine will be (will look like cola).

- Drink regularly or whenever possible during workouts and operations. Drink 12–18 oz of fluid every 20 minutes to maintain hydration;

- Weigh yourself before and after an event to determine how much fluid is lost.

- Every one pound of weight lost requires 125–150% more fluid or 20–24 oz. It will take about 6 hours to recover from dehydration post exercise/ military operation.

- Performance decrements begin when only 2% of body weight has been lost.

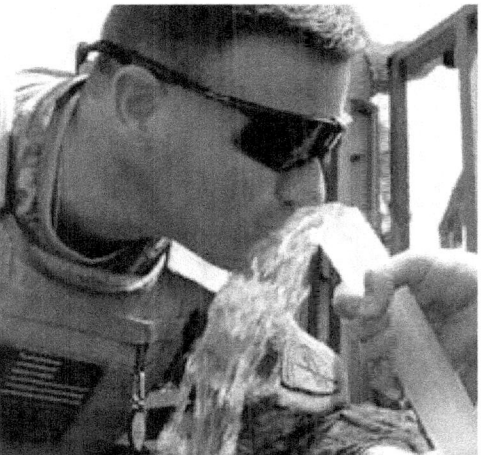

What Should You Drink?

Although the type of activity will determine what to drink, the beverage selected should:

- Empty from your stomach and intestines rapidly.

- Taste good.

- Provide CHO when exercise lasts > 1 hr.

- Contain a small amount of sodium (salt).

- Provide no more than 19 grams of CHO per 8 oz.

- Be cool (10 to 15°C).

- Be diluted to ≤ 9 grams CHO/8 oz or a 4–5% CHO solution if fluid needs are > 4L.

Fluid Replacement Beverages

If the exercise is longer than one hour, a beverage that provides CHO should be ingested. Beverages with "glucose polymers" (maltodextrin), or a mixture of glucose and fructose are usually preferable to glucose or sucrose alone. The important message is "drink." A list of beverages, some of which are used as "fluid replacement beverages" by athletes, and a set of criteria for selecting commercial off-the-shelf fluids replacement beverages are presented in Table 3–7.

Fluid replacement beverages that contain more than 19 grams of CHO per 8 oz may cause stomach distress and not be absorbed well if consumed before or during physical activity. For example, orange juice should be mixed with an equal amount of water because it is so concentrated.

Criteria for Commercial Off-The-Shelf Fluid Replacement Beverages

- < 95 kcal/8oz.

- CHO Content: 9–19 g/8oz.

- CHO to Protein Ratio: > 4:1 ratio, if any protein/amino acids.

- Sodium: 0.2–1.15 g/L (40-240 mg/8 oz).

- No carbonation.

- No substances other than CHO, electrolytes, and protein.

Table 3–7. Commercial Off-The-Shelf Fluid Replacement Beverages Meeting Criteria				
Products	Energy kcal/8 oz	CHO g/8 oz	CHO:Pro ≥ 4:1	Sodium mg/8oz
CarboPack Beverage	94	19	-	55–160
Cerasport	76	13	-	102
Gatorade Original	50	14	-	110
Gookinade	86	10	-	64
GU2O	50	13	-	120
MetRx ORS	75	19	-	125

Products	Energy kcal/8 oz	CHO g/8 oz	CHO:Pro ≥ 4:1	Sodium mg/8oz
Powerade	72	19	-	53
Power Bar Endurance Sports Drink	70	17	-	160
Gatorade Endurance	50	14	-	200

Table 3–7. Commercial Off-The-Shelf Fluid Replacement Beverages Meeting Criteria

When and How Much to Drink?

Remember: although the following recommendations are generally sound for most people, everyone is different. Each person must learn to look for signs alerting to his fluid needs. Make adjustments to how warm/hot it is outside. If very hot, make sure to drink fluids with sodium to replace lost electrolytes from sweating. The more physical activity, the more fluid needed! Be careful not to drink **too** much plain water, especially during prolonged exercise in the heat. The figure to the right shows daily water requirements as a function of activity and environmental temperature.

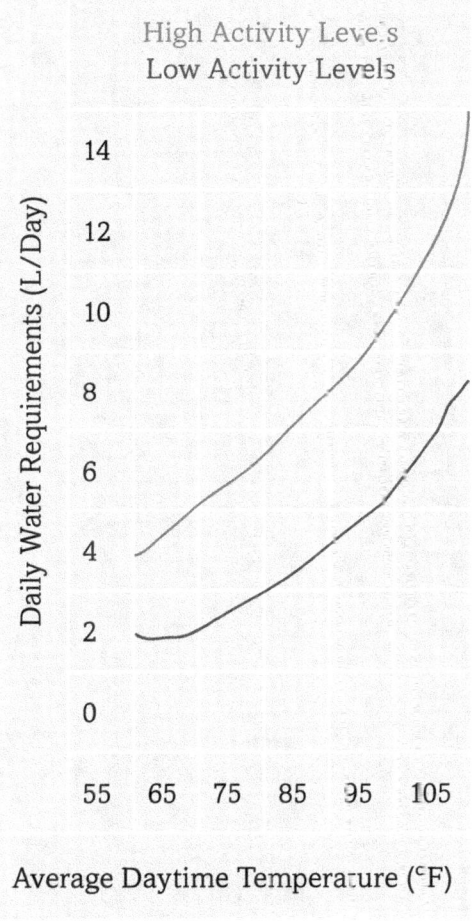

High Activity Levels
Low Activity Levels

Daily Water Requirements (L/Day)

Average Daytime Temperature (°F)

"A Warfighter needs the right nutrition and quantity of food in the same way a high performance car needs the right mixture of high octane fuel and air to achieve peak performance."

CDR Todd L. Tinsley, NSWSBT22

4 High Performance Catalysts

In This Chapter

Role of High Performance Catalysts in WF

Dietary Reference Intakes and Definitions

Nutrient Density

Vitamins

Minerals

Special Catalysts: Antioxidants

Substances That Interfere with High Performance Catalysts

Vitamin & Mineral Dietary Supplements

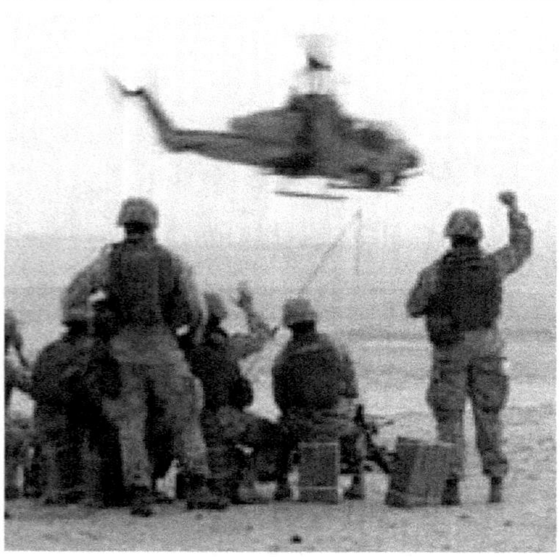

Key Points

- Vitamin and mineral needs can be met by eating a variety of foods.
- Vitamin-mineral supplements do not provide energy.
- Vitamin-mineral supplementation is warranted only when energy balance is not met through the diet.
- Mega-dosing on vitamins and minerals can be detrimental to health and performance.
- Foods naturally high in antioxidants (fresh and colorful foods) should be eaten daily.

High performance catalysts, or micronutrients, allow performance at a high level. Catalysts include vitamins, minerals, and other essential nutrients required by the body in very small amounts to perform vital metabolic and physiologic functions. Taking in too little or too much of these nutrients can interfere with normal body functions.

Role of High Performance Catalysts in Warfighters

Some of functions of high performance catalysts are presented below.

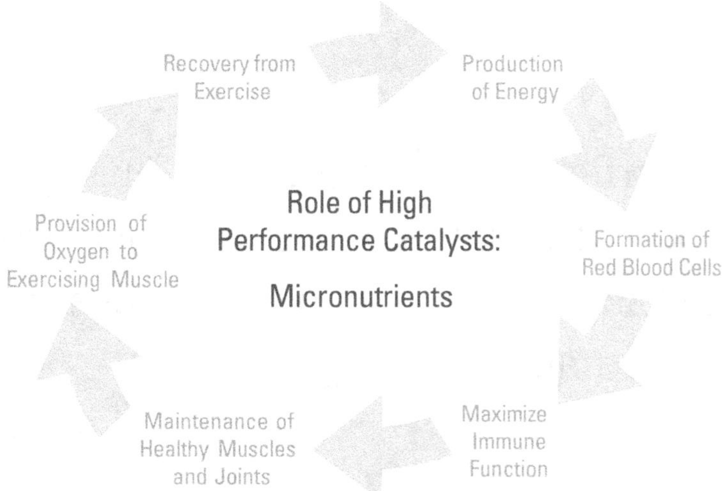

Recovery from Exercise
Production of Energy
Formation of Red Blood Cells
Maximize Immune Function
Maintenance of Healthy Muscles and Joints
Provision of Oxygen to Exercising Muscle
Role of High Performance Catalysts:
Micronutrients

> If energy intake is sufficient, the high catalyst requirements of Warfighters should be adequate.

Different amounts of catalysts are needed by individuals, depending on gender, age, activity, and environment. The best way to obtain the required amounts is to eat well-balanced meals with foods that are nutrient dense. A daily diet of diverse foods can provide the necessary amounts of high performance catalysts for a well-tuned body.

Dietary Reference Intakes and Definitions

Various terms have been developed to explain how much of these "catalysts" are needed. The term **Dietary Reference Intakes** (DRI's) refers to the amount of particular vitamins and minerals a typical person should eat to prevent a deficiency. The DRIs also have a **Tolerable Upper Intake Level** (ULs) that tells us how much is *too* much. The term % **Daily Value** (DV) on a food label represents how much one serving contributes nutritionally to a 2,000-calorie-a-day diet. If the label says 15% DV for Vitamin C, then one serving provides 15% of the DRI for Vitamin C. Other terms and definitions are noted on the side bar.

The U.S. Military also has **Military Dietary Reference Intakes** (MDRIs) based on the U.S. DRIs. They are for planning, assessing diets, and developing rations for the military population. Neither DRIs or MDRIs consider the nutrient needs of Warfighters, who train and operate under diverse, often grueling, environmental conditions.

Nutrient Density

The term "nutrient density" is important to understand. It is the amount of a particular nutrient (vitamin, mineral, carbohydrate, protein, fat, etc.) per unit of energy in a given food, or per gram of food. It is also an index of nutritional quality. In the following table, Comparison 1 shows the nutrient density of the food label for granola versus glazed donuts. Comparison 2 shows the information for orange juice versus coca cola. The granola and orange juice are clearly more "nutrient dense" than their comparative foods.

Table 4–1. Examples and Comparisons of Nutrient Density			
Comparison 1		**Comparison 2**	
Kashi Go Lean Crunch (1 oz)	**Glazed Donut (1 oz)**	**Orange Juice (100 ml)**	**Coca Cola (100 ml)**
0% DV for Vitamin A	0% DV for Vitamin A	4% DV for Vitamin A	0% DV for Vitamin A

Table 4–1. Examples and Comparisons of Nutrient Density			
Comparison 1		**Comparison 2**	
Kashi Go Lean Crunch (1 oz)	**Glazed Donut (1 oz)**	**Orange Juice (100 ml)**	**Coca Cola (100 ml)**
3% DV for Calcium	1% DV for Calcium	1% DV for Calcium	0% DV for Calcium
0% DV for Vitamin C	0% DV for Vitamin C	83% DV for Vitamin C	0% DV for Vitamin C
5% DV for Iron	3% DV for Iron	1% DV for Iron	0% DV for Iron
20 g Fiber	0 g Fiber	0 g Fiber	0 g Fiber
10 g Protein	1 g Protein	1 g Protein	0 g Protein

Many other examples could be presented, but clearly foods with more fiber, "high performance catalysts," and less fat and simple sugars should be selected. At least 90% of the diet should be comprised of nutrient dense foods.

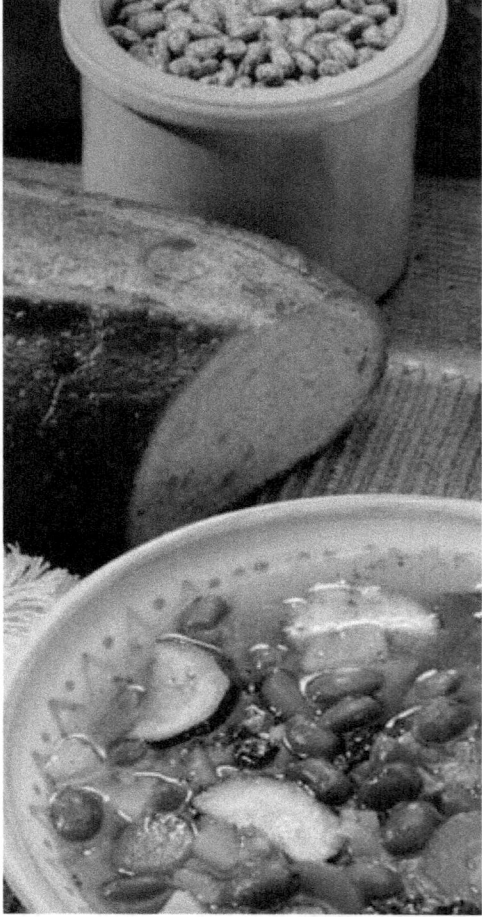

Vitamins

Vitamins are organic compounds that allow for energy to be produced, among other functions. They are broadly classified as water- and fat-soluble: water-soluble vitamins dissolve in water and are not stored, but rather eliminated through urine; therefore, a continuous supply is needed in the

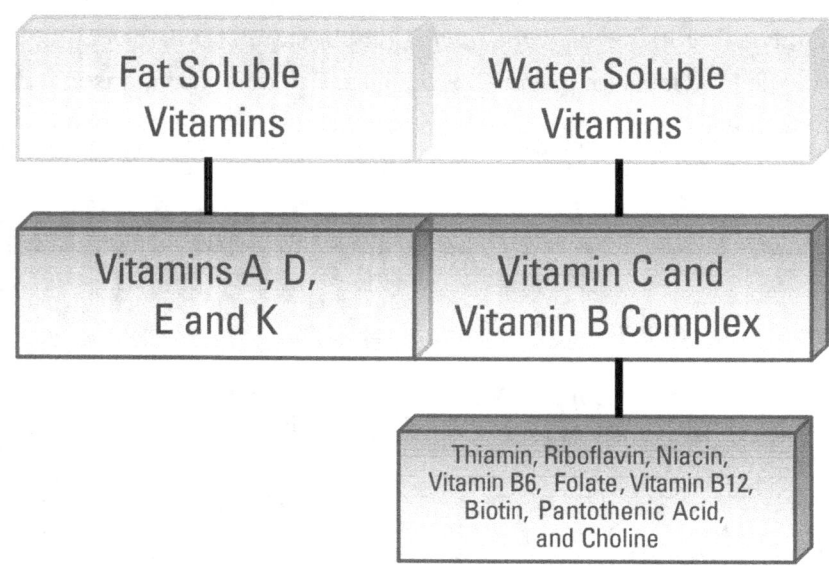

diet. However, fat-soluble vitamins are not required every day because they are stored in fat tissue and the liver. Fat-soluble vitamins are best absorbed with dietary fat. Choline is another essential nutrient and similar to the B-vitamins, but not officially listed as a B-vitamin.

Functions of Vitamins

- Production of energy from macronutrients (CHO, fats, and proteins).
- Repair and growth of tissue.
- Maintenance and support of reproductive function.
- Development of immune response.

Some functions may be specific to only one vitamin, whereas other functions may require more than one vitamin. For example, several B vitamins and some minerals are required to produce energy from foods.

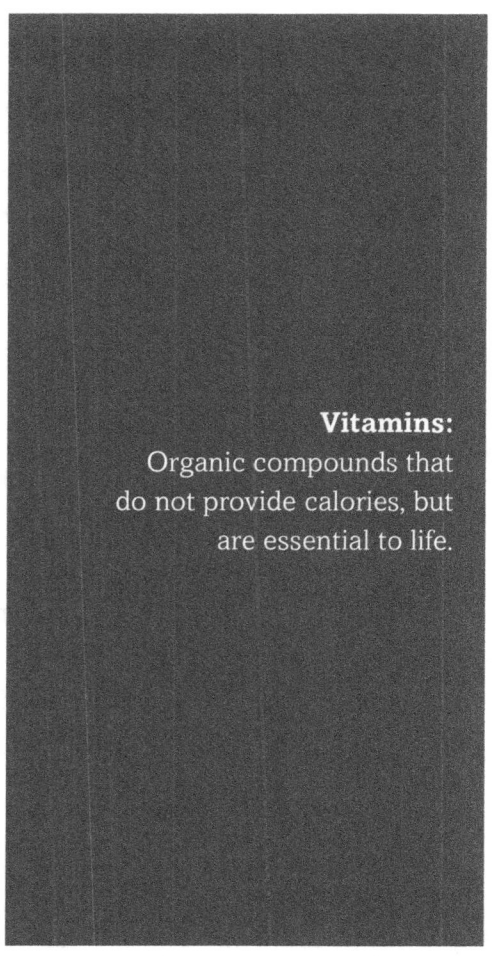

Vitamins:
Organic compounds that do not provide calories, but are essential to life.

Good Food Sources of Vitamins

No single food is a good source of all vitamins, which is why it is important to eat a variety of foods. Some processed foods provide many vitamins because they have been fortified with nutrients, whereas other foods may contain few, if any, vitamins. When eating at home or dining away from home, the key to eating a balanced meal is choosing a variety of foods, whenever possible. To obtain the necessary vitamins, a dinner plate should include:

- A heaping pile of vegetables (excluding potatoes and corn).
- Black, pinto, or kidney beans and whole grains or corn.
- Fish, lean poultry, or lean cuts of red meat, tofu, dairy products.
- Nuts/seeds.

If eating field rations during training or deployment, eat the entrees as well as the other food and beverage items provided in the pack since different food/beverage items are fortified with different micronutrients. For example, cocoa in the Meal Ready to Eat ration is a source of vitamin B1, calcium and magnesium.

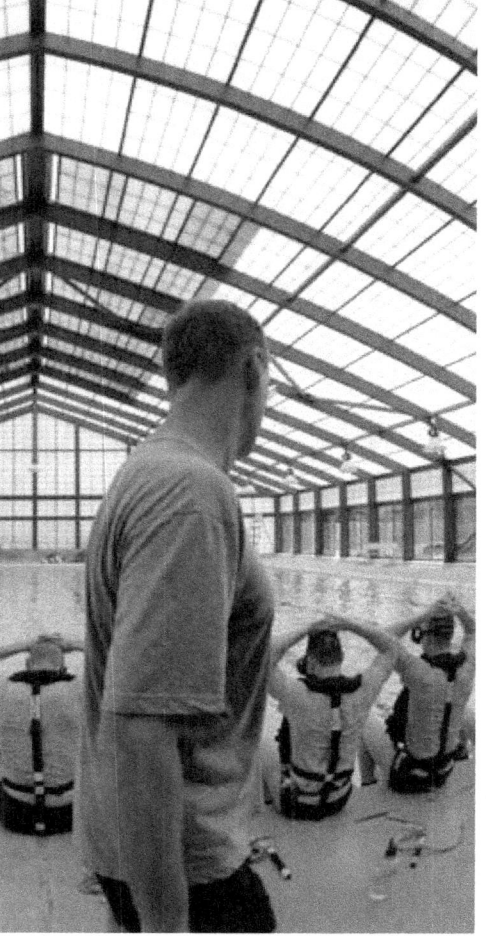

Preserving Vitamins in Foods

Proper food storage and preparation can minimize vitamin losses. All vitamins are destroyed by light and many are destroyed by excessive heat. Water-soluble vitamins are easily washed out when foods are over-cooked. Steps that should be taken to increase the retention of vitamins during storage and preparation include:

- Keep foods out of direct light as much as possible, especially milk and grains.

- Keep fresh produce refrigerated.

- Avoid soaking vegetables in water.

- Cook in just enough water to prevent burning.

- Use the shortest cooking time by cooking to a crisp and tender stage.

- Steaming and stir frying result in the best vitamin retention.

- Cut and cook vegetables shortly before serving or refrigerate in an airtight storage container.

Minerals

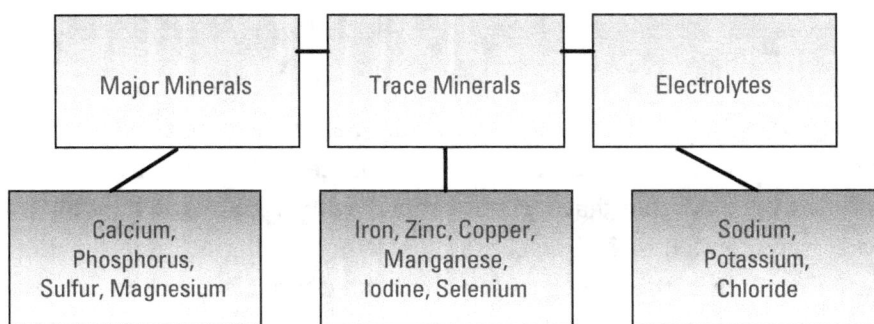

Minerals are inorganic substances that can be single elements, such as magnesium (Mg) and calcium (Ca), simple salts (electrolytes), or metals, such as iron (Fe). Numerous minerals are required by the body, and may account for 4–5% of a person's body weight. Typically, minerals are classified as major minerals, trace minerals, or electrolytes, depending on function and how much is in the body.

Major minerals are required in relatively large amounts (> 200 mg/day), whereas **trace minerals** are required in smaller amounts (< 200 mg/day). They can occur naturally in food or be added in elemental or mineral form. Appropriate dietary intakes of minerals must be sustained to maintain physical health. Excessive intakes may lead to adverse consequences because of the competitive nature between minerals in the body. For example, zinc and copper, and calcium and magnesium are needed in particular ratios. Electrolytes include sodium, potassium, and chloride.

Functions of Minerals

- Brain and neural function.

- Bone structure and maintenance.

Minerals:
Inorganic compounds found in all body tissues and essential for life.

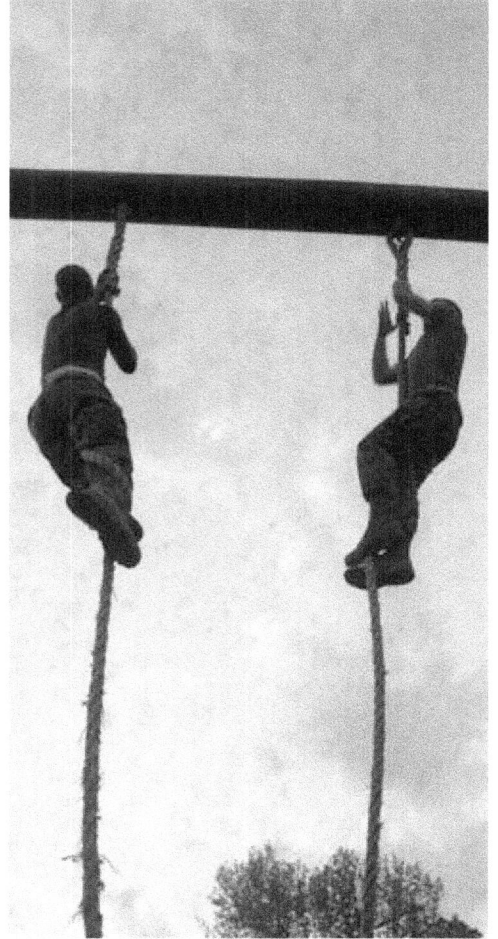

- Muscle function and growth.

- Production of energy.

- Reproductive functions.

- Immune function.

Good Food Sources of Minerals

As with vitamins, a variety of foods should be eaten in order to meet requirements for these essential nutrients. Table 4–2 provides a list of foods that are high in selected minerals.

Table 4–2. Primary Food Sources for Some Minerals	
Food Products	**Major Mineral**
Green leafy vegetables and dairy products	Calcium
Nuts, soy beans, and cocoa	Magnesium
Milk and spinach	Sodium
Legumes, whole grains, and bananas	Potassium
Table salt	Chloride, iodine
Meat, eggs, and legumes	Sulfur
Red meat, poultry and seafood	Zinc
Red meat and leafy vegetables	Iron

Mineral Requirements for Military Garrison Training

The MDRIs reflect the Institute of Medicine (IOM) Dietary Reference Intakes (DRIs). Modifications to these requirements should only be made when sufficient scientific evidence exists to support different requirements and intakes. The recommended values for some minerals should take into account enhanced mineral losses caused by high-performance activities.

Evidence strongly indicates that sweat mineral losses of copper, iron and zinc might be significant during garrison training. New recommendations reflect this evidence (See Table 4–3). However, insufficient data exists for sweat losses of calcium, magnesium and selenium to recommend an increased intake. Also, requirements might be different for specific military situations and more research is required prior to changing current recommendations.

Table 4–3. Mineral Intakes for Men: Institute of Medicine Dietary Reference Intakes, Current Military Dietary Reference Intakes, and Recommended Levels for Military Garrison Training and Assault Rations				
Nutrient	IOM RDA or AI*	MDRI	RDA of AI for MGT	RDA for Assault Rations*
Calcium (mg)	1,000	1,000	1,000	750–850
Copper (µg)	900	ND	1,800	900–1,600
Iron (mg)	8	10	14	8–18
Magnesium (mg)	420	420	420	400–550
Selenium (µg)	55	55	55	55–230
Zinc (mg)	11	15	15	11–25

Note: Institute of Medicine = IOM; RDA= Recommended Dietary Allowance; AI=Adequate Intake; MDRI = Military Dietary Reference Intakes; MGT= Military Garrison Training; ND= Not Determined; *Institute of Medicine (2006).

Special Catalysts: Antioxidants

Antioxidants are substances in foods that neutralize highly reactive, destructive compounds called free radicals. Note the following key points about free radicals and antioxidants:

- Free radical damage can lead to cancer and heart disease.

- Free radicals from harmful pollutants are neutralized by antioxidants.

- Foods rich in antioxidants are the best source of antioxidants.

- Smokers should consume foods high in antioxidants.

Some well known antioxidants include:

- Vitamin E.
- Selenium.

- Beta Carotene.
- Glutathione.

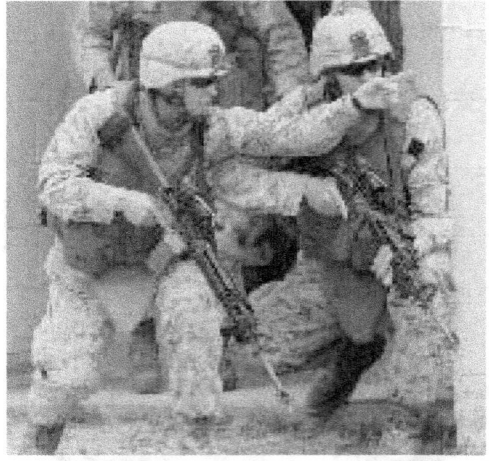

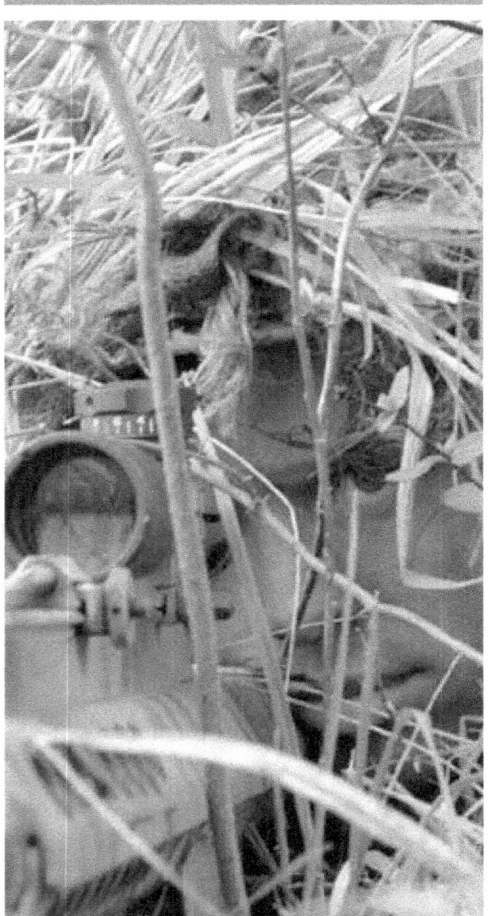

- Cysteine.
- Vitamin C.
- Flavonoids.
- Glutathione.

Some critical antioxidants are enzymes, such as superoxide dismutase, and catalase. Additional antioxidant details are discussed in Chapter 18.

Antioxidants should come from food.

Substances That Interfere With High Performance Catalysts

Many substances affect both the absorption and loss of high performance catalysts. For example, the amount absorbed from foods can be influenced by dietary constituents (such as fiber), other factors (such as medications), the body's need for the nutrient, the chemical form of the nutrient, and the integrity of the digestive tract. "ANTI-catalysts" that can interfere with how well the body uses nutrients are shown below:

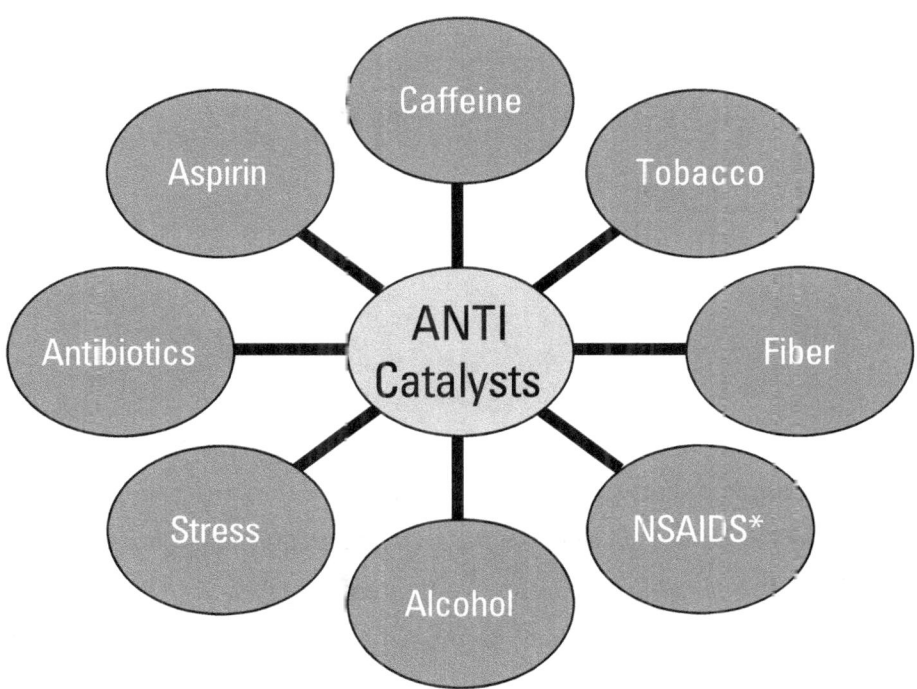

*Nonsteroidal Anti-Inflammatory Drugs

To minimize the potential effects of ANTI-catalysts, one should:

- Eat a variety of foods.
- Use good food preparation techniques.

Vitamin and Mineral Dietary Supplements

The DRI for high performance catalysts provide a wide safety margin, but some adjustments may be required in individuals with very high energy expenditures. Nutrient requirements for antioxidant vitamins (C, E and carotenoids), B vitamins, magnesium, zinc, copper, selenium and iron needs may be slightly higher in Warfighters because of activity levels. But, a good, varied diet will allow the DRI to be met. Despite this, the supplement industry encourages physically active people to purchase vitamin and mineral supplements to enhance performance. About 40–80% of military personnel use some form of vitamin and/or mineral supplements. These include single vitamins (vitamin C), minerals (calcium) and/or multivitamin-mineral combinations. In many cases the doses range from amounts similar to or far in excess of the DRI. Vitamin and mineral supplements are useful when:

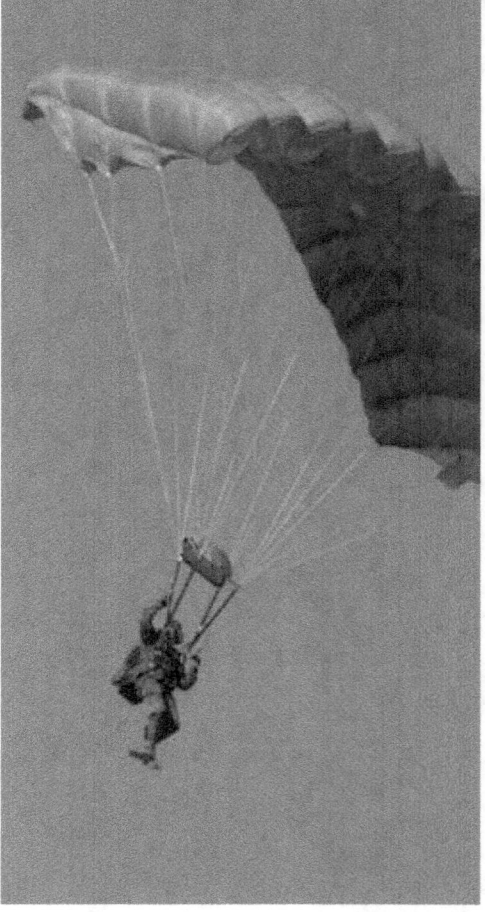

- An existing vitamin or mineral deficiency is present.

- Individuals have poor nutrient intakes and dietary habits.

- Energy requirements cannot be met by food.

- Individuals are exposed to extreme environments, such as strenuous exercise, cold exposure, and at high altitude.

Vitamin and Mineral Supplement Use and Performance

Taking a general multivitamin/mineral supplement appears to be without measurable performance benefit in healthy, well-nourished, physically active men. Whether supplementation with such nutrients produces beneficial effects on performance in Warfighters is unknown. For example, supplementation with selected vitamins/minerals may accelerate recovery or reduce susceptibility to infections. Some information to confirm these possibilities is available, but studies have not been conducted in military populations. If a vitamin and/or mineral supplement is desired, the supplement should provide nutrients in amounts that meet the DRI, and no supplement should provide more than the Upper Limit as indicated by the National Academy of Sciences.

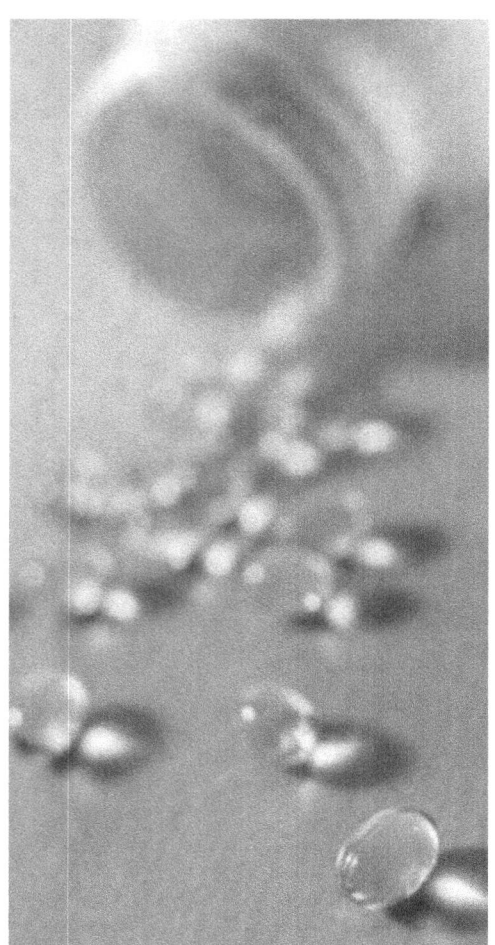

The illustration below presents the relative amounts of "popular" vitamin and minerals needed on a daily basis.

Relative Daily Intake of Vitamins and Minerals (mg/d)

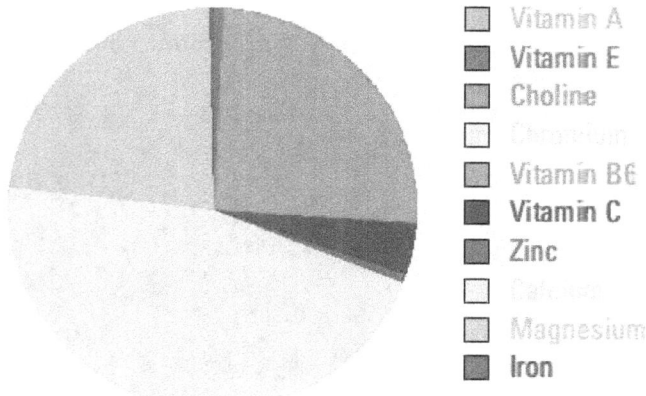

- Vitamin A
- Vitamin E
- Choline
- Chromium
- Vitamin B6
- Vitamin C
- Zinc
- Calcium
- Magnesium
- Iron

Risks of Vitamin and Mineral Supplements

Excessive intakes of some vitamin and mineral supplements can cause multiple side effects, and some vitamins and minerals can be toxic. Although some people take excessive amounts of nutrients on a regular basis, it is important to distinguish between excessive and toxic. Excessive amounts of single or multiple nutrient supplements can upset overall nutrient balance and cause a deficiency of other nutrients. Iron, zinc and copper are good examples, since all three are absorbed via the same route. An excessive intake of zinc can prevent the proper absorption of the others. Additionally, excess vitamin E (in the form of alpha tocopherol) has been shown to slow healing, inhibit the immune system, and increase the risk of bleeding. Symptoms may include fatigue, weakness, headache, blurred vision, and diarrhea. Other fat-soluble vitamins, such as vitamin A and D, can also be taken in excess. Vitamin C overdoses are unlikely, but taking a lot of vitamin C followed by low levels can lead to "rebound scurvy." Importantly, intakes above DRI upper limits may have significant adverse effects. Table 4–4 provides a list of various nutrients and levels considered to be toxic.

To avoid harmful effects from high doses of supplemental vitamins and minerals, refer to the DRI upper limits.

Vitamin and mineral supplements are absorbed best when taken with food.

Table 4–4. Nutrients and Their Toxicity Values			
Nutrient	Toxicity (units/day)	Nutrient	Toxicity (units/day)
Vitamin A	>25,000 IU	Magnesium	>6,000 mg
Beta Carotene	None	Boron	>100 mg

Table 4–4. Nutrients and Their Toxicity Values			
Nutrient	**Toxicity (units/day)**	**Nutrient**	**Toxicity (units/day)**
Vitamin D	>50,000 IU	Chromium	>10 mg
Vitamin E	>1,200 IU	Copper	>35 mg
Vitamin B6	>2,000 mg	Iron	>100 mg
Vitamin C	Rare	Selenium	>1 mg
Calcium	>2,500 mg	Zinc	>150 mg

Do not take a vitamin/mineral supplement with a carbohydrate-protein drink that already contains vitamins and minerals or the supplement and money will be wasted: excess amounts are excreted in the urine.

5 Nutrient Timing and Training

Key Points

- The timing of nutrient delivery is critical to sustaining performance.

- The **Refueling Interval (RFI)** is the 45 minutes after finishing a workout.

- Eating during the RFI will accelerate recovery and restore energy for the next day's workout.

- A daily diet that is balanced and nutrient-dense will ensure better performance and optimal recovery.

- CHO foods and beverages that have a moderate to high glycemic index, such as sport drinks, raisins, honey, bananas or potatoes are ideal recovery foods.

- Adding protein to the recovery meal will help stimulate protein synthesis to assist in rebuilding muscle (anabolism).

- For exercise longer than 90 minutes, consume 50 grams of CHO and 12 grams of protein as food and/or drink during the RFI. Then ingest about 50 grams of CHO every hour for up to 6 hours, depending on duration of exercise.

- Adequate fluids must be ingested after a mission.

- Fluid replacement beverages should contain sodium and potassium.

- Sports bars, gels and drinks are lightweight, portable and easy to eat during military operations.

The goals of training are to promote changes in the body such that muscular strength, aerobic capacity, and endurance are optimized. Training goals cannot be achieved in the absence of appropriate nutritional strategies. Before and after training or missions, strategies to ensure adequate energy stores and rapid recovery for the next mission are critical. Well conceived meal and snack plans will enhance preparedness, boost morale, stimulate muscle protein synthesis, and help protect against training injuries. Nutrient timing combined with rest are essential. This chapter will provide information about nutritional strategies to optimize training in preparation for missions.

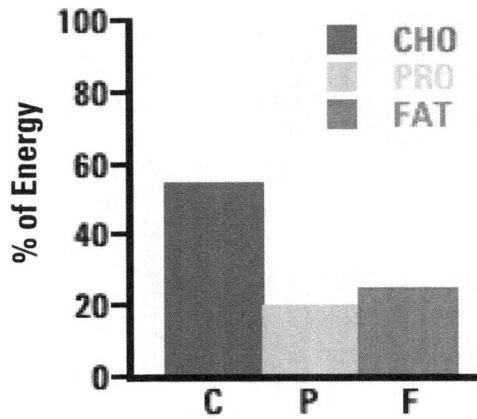

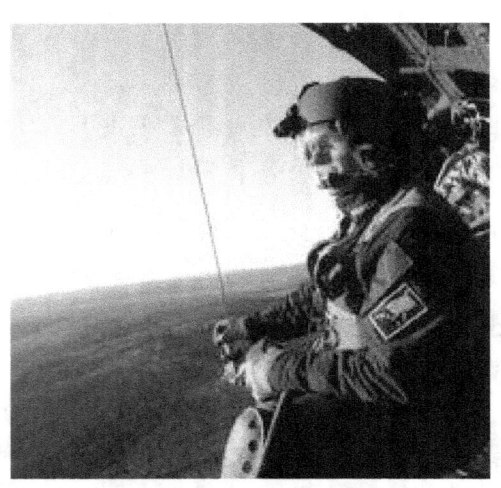

Warfighter Activity:
Recall an operation that caused complete fatigue as a result of sustained effort for mission success.

Everyday Nutrition and the "ine" Diet

For performance and recovery to be optimal, the everyday diet of Warfighters must be as good as it possibly can be. Routine dietary habits must be considered to determine what should be done to ensure operational performance and overall good health. The usual CPF (CHO: Protein: Fat) pattern should approximate: CHO—55%; Protein—20%; and Fat—25%. This is not the usual Warfighter pattern.

Navy SEAL Mike Fullerton stated that all military members are on the so called "**ine diet.**" "We all wake up at 0-dark thirty, grab a big gulp of java (caff**eine**), dip a pinch of Skoal (nicot**ine**) and grab a few honey buns from the "gee-dunk" (vending mach**ine**)." This pattern of eating over many years comes back with revenge, and makes recovery from strenuous missions more and more difficult. The following other dietary practices are admitted by many Warfighters:

- Consuming the majority of calories at the end of the day.

- Underestimating calories consumed and portions eaten.

- Planning meals poorly.

- Eating too much fast food chow.

- Using multiple dietary supplements to enhance performance.

- Using caffeine and simple sugars to fill the void during the day.

The following operations require nutritional countermeasures to avoid complete exhaustion and muscular fatigue:

- Wearing boots and body armor and carrying heavy packs and ammunitions for over 60 minutes.

- Fast roping or dragging a wounded comrade to safety.

- Extended water operations.

- Altitude operations.

- Prolonged shivering in austere environments, such as operating in mountainous regions or diving in cold water.

Fatigue and Glycogen Depletion

Fatigue is a complex phenomenon caused by failure at multiple sites during exercise. The causes of fatigue can be central (mind/central nervous system or neuromuscular) and/or local (peripheral—muscle). One nutritional cause of fatigue is depletion of muscle glycogen. All strenuous exercise, be it endurance, resistance training or missions, will deplete glycogen. Muscle glycogen must be replenished through nutritional interventions to override fatigue and accelerate recovery.

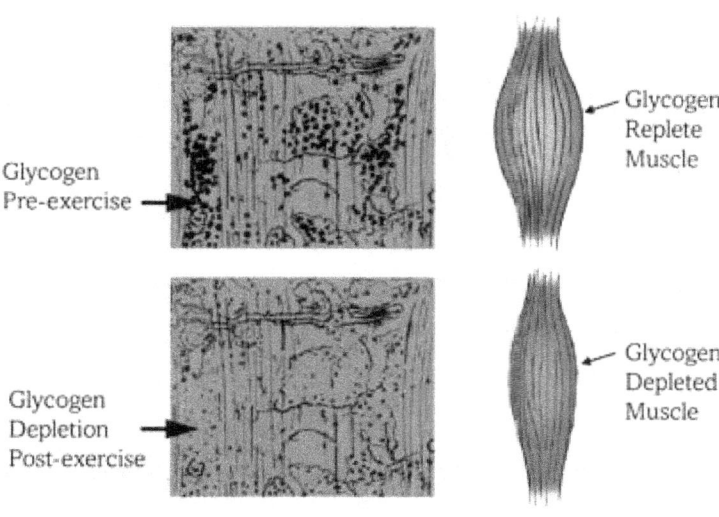

Glycogen Pre-exercise

Glycogen Depletion Post-exercise

Glycogen Replete Muscle

Glycogen Depleted Muscle

It takes at least 24 hours to replenish muscle glycogen stores following exhaustive exercise or operations.

Glycogen repletion occurs when enough CHO is provided. If diet is neglected over time, "staleness" can become a problem.

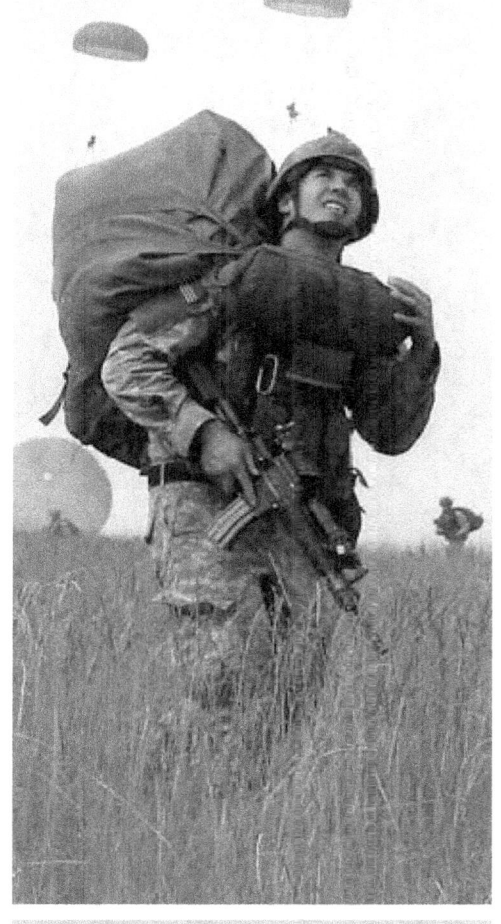

"Staleness" and Overtraining

The terms "staleness and "overtraining" are consistently noted for competitive athletes and may apply to Warfighters as well. Staleness and/or overtraining are believed to result from too little recovery time in combination with too much training. Other factors or non-training stressors can also contribute to staleness. A multitude of symptoms are associated with overtraining, including:

• Unexplained, persistently poor performance.

• Moodiness, general fatigue, depression, and irritability.

• Painful muscles.

• Elevated morning resting pulse.

• Insomnia.

• Weight loss.

• Overuse injuries.

• Increased susceptibility to upper respiratory infections and gut problems.

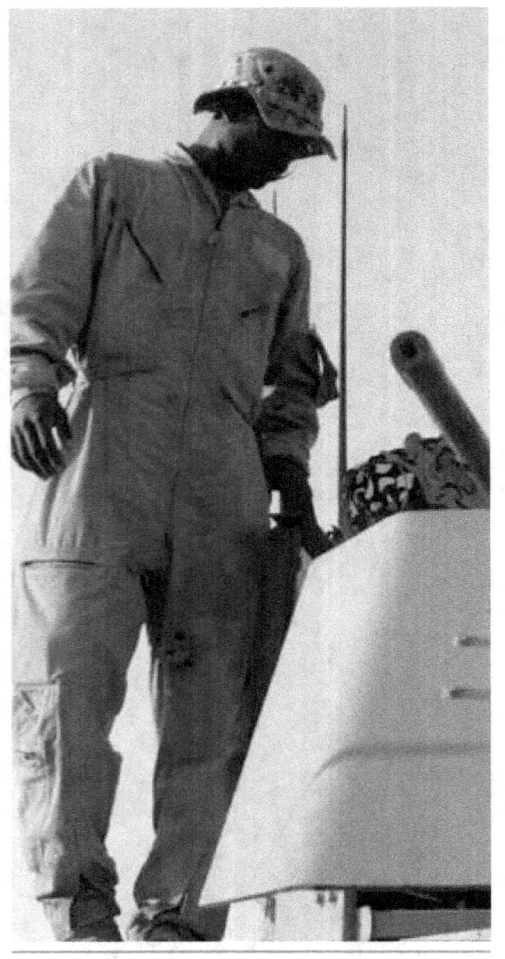

Too rigorous a training program can impair immune function.

How staleness or overtraining is expressed depends upon the physical and physiological makeup of the warrior, type of training regimens, dietary practices, sleep patterns, and various other factors. No single test can identify overtraining, but a number of key markers that change over time have been proposed. Possible markers include stress hormones, immune markers, indicators of muscle damage, compromised muscle glycogen reserves, and decrements in aerobic and anaerobic capacity. Drs. Jack Raglin and William Morgan from Indiana University developed a scale to identify endurance athletes who exhibit signs of distress resulting from intensive training. Called the Training Distress Scale, it consists of ten items that are individually scored and then used to create a total score. If an individual's total score is high over several consecutive days, a couple of days of rest are critical to preserve future performance.

The Remedy

CHO intake over 24 hours will typically not exceed 650 grams.

- Make sure that training is accompanied by periods of rest.

- Ingest a meal providing 2 grams of CHO per pound of body weight approximately 4 hours prior to exercise.

- Ingest 0.4 grams of a low GI CHO drink or solid food per pound of body weight 1 hour before exercise.

- Consume an easily digested, high-CHO drink or food that provides approximately 50 grams of CHO and 12 grams of protein within 45 minutes after exercise.

- Consume 0.5 grams of CHO per pound of body weight, or at least 50 grams, every 60 minutes for up to 6 hours after exercise, depending on exercise intensity and duration.

- Consume a high CHO drink or solid food providing at least 250 kcal (60 grams) of CHO with each meal.

- Be certain your body weight is stable during all phases of training by matching energy intake to energy requirements.

Example: CHO in grams for a 155 lb warrior:

Before Exercise:

233 g (155 x 1.5) of CHO 4 hrs before
62 g (155 x 0.4) of a low GI CHO up to 1 hr before

Immediately After Exercise:

50 g of CHO and 12 grams of protein
1–4 hours after exercise
78 g (155 x 0.5) of CHO every 30 minutes until 4 hrs

Table 5–1. CHO Content (grams) of Various Foods and Beverages	
Low-fat milk, 1 cup	12
Bread, 1 slice	13
Oatmeal cookie, 1	15
Pound cake, 1 slice	15
Apple, 1	19
Blueberries, 1 cup	20
Wheaties, 1 cup	25
Blueberry muffin, 1	25
Pear, 1	25
Baked potato, 1	25
Bean & meat burrito, 1	33
Banana, 1	35
Sweet corn, 1 cup	40
Macaroni, 1 cup	40
Rice, 1 cup	40
Cinnamon bagel, 4"	50
Bagged pretzels, 10	50
Pancakes & syrup, 2	90
Seedless raisins, 1 cup	130

Nutrient Timing

The timing of "when" nutrients are consumed may be as important as "what" nutrients are consumed.

The timing of nutrients should be viewed as three very distinct phases:

- Recovery or maintenance.

- Exercise when energy stores are being depleted.

- The RFI, or critical period after exercise.

During exercise the environment is "catabolic" so that energy can be delivered to the working muscles. Insulin, an important hormone for promoting muscle protein synthesis, is not released during exercise because it is not needed. After exercise the environments must become "anabolic," so the process of recovery and building up what was lost begins: insulin

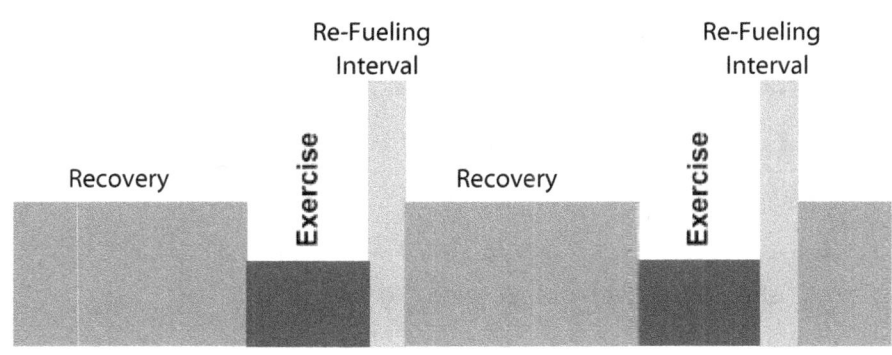

Phases of Timing Nutrient Intake

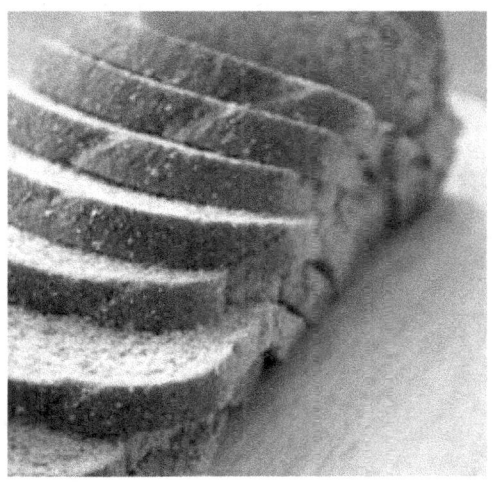

Nutritional intervention within 45 minutes after exercise is the most critical time, or "RFI," for recovery.

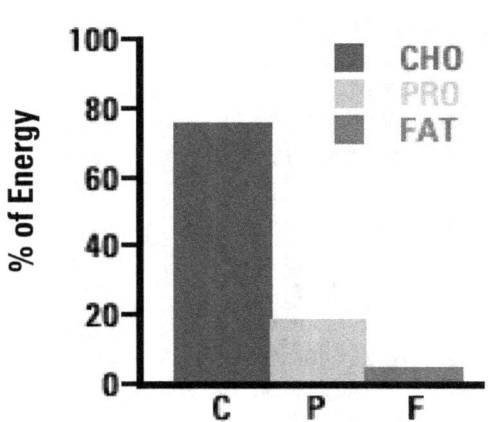

release must be stimulated. Ingestion of CHO stimulates "insulin." Thus, immediately after exercise, when glycogen stores and muscle protein synthesis are low, is the critical time to provide what the body or muscle needs: CHO with a small amount of protein.

Running on an empty tank for too long after strenuous operations or PT will be detrimental to performance and duties the next day. To avoid performance decrements, or fatigue, a CPF of 80%/20%/0%, or as little fat as possible, is recommended. This means a small meal of CHO (50–60 grams) and protein (12–15 grams), taken as food or fluid within 45 minutes after completing exercise, will help begin repletion of muscle glycogen stores and synthesis of muscle protein. This RFI will set the stage for both recovery, repair, and muscular growth.

RFI: Consume 50 g of CHO and 12 g of protein within 45 minutes after training.

More protein may compromise recovery and muscle protein synthesis.

Glycemic Index:

Describes how a particular food raises blood glucose levels.

☀ List of Glycemic Index Classification.

Table 5–2. Possible RFI Foods		
Food and/or Beverage Product(s)	CHO (g)	Protein (g)
Peanut butter, 2 Tbsp, and jelly, 2 tsp, on wheat bread, 2 slices	43	14
Wendy's Mandarin Chicken Salad and Cran-apple juice, 8 oz	88	27
Hard-boiled egg, 1, and bagel	56	12
Hand-Tossed Style Chicken Supreme Pizza (Pizza Hut), 1 slice, and juice, 8 oz	57	13
McDonald English Muffins with Jam, 2	36	5
Subway Oatmeal Raisin Cookie and 6" Deli Turkey Breast Sub	76	21
Subway Breakfast Western Egg with Cheese on Deli Roll with orange juice, 4 oz	43	0
Taco Bell Bean Burrito, 1	54	13

Table 5–2. Possible RFI Foods		
Food and/or Beverage Product(s)	CHO (g)	Protein (g)
Low-fat yogurt with fruit, 8 oz	47	11
Soldier Fuel Bar, 1, or other high CHO Sports Bar	40	10
String cheese, 2, and apple or pear, 1 large	23	14
Cereal with low-fat milk, 1 cup	53	13
Arby's Jamocha Shake, regular size	81	11

Good food choices should be made throughout the recovery/maintenance phase when muscle growth and tissue repair are needed.

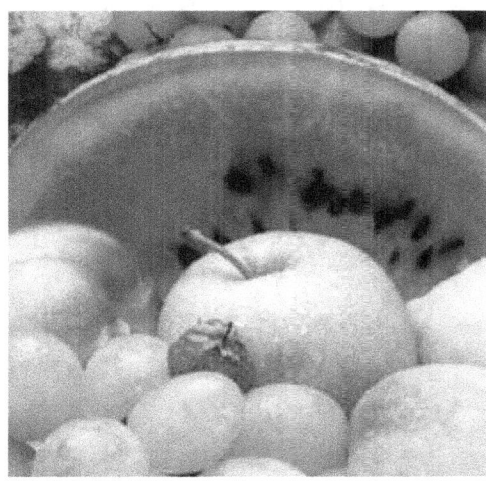

After the first 45 minutes, nutrient intake will depend on the duration, intensity, and type of activity. Low intensity exercise of short duration will require regular meals at regular intervals, whereas high intensity exercise of both short and long duration will require regular snacks of carbohydrate and protein, with some fat. Obviously, the longer the duration of the activity, the greater the energy drain, thus a greater need for refueling the tank.

A recovery meal to ensure nutrients, fluids, and calories are replenished immediately after PT during the RFI and over the course of the day is important. Examples of nutrient-dense recovery foods include the following:

- Sports bar, 1, with 50 g CHO and 12 g protein.

- 100% fruit juice, 8 oz.

- Low-fat yogurt, 8 oz.

- Whole grain bagel, 1.

- Honey, 1 oz.

- Cottage cheese, 4 oz.

- Tuna fish, 3 oz.

- Tomato or V8 juice, 8 oz.

- Whole fruit, 1 piece.

- Homemade trail mix, 6 oz.

These Recovery Meals ensure that nutrient-dense foods, to include carbohydrate-rich, high quality protein, and healthy fats are eaten by War-fighters at the right time. Commercial Off the Shelf (COTS) products are being used in some military commands currently to help provide carbo-hydrate-rich foods such as sports drinks, bars, and gels during training so

they can train and deploy with the same products. These nutrition initiatives have allowed Warfighters to access nutritionally desirable foods within their commands immediately after PT and in operational settings. Most importantly, COTS are considered "comfort foods" because they are familiar and previously used during phases of training.

All Carbohydrates are NOT Created Equally

Not all CHO foods are equally effective in restoring blood glucose. Certain foods raise blood glucose concentrations and promote glycogen synthesis better than others. The term Glycemic Index is used to describe (and rank) how high a particular food will raise blood glucose; foods with a high glycemic index (GI) are the most effective for restoring glycogen. As shown in the graph, a high GI food produces a "spike" in blood glucose, whereas a low GI food takes a longer time to peak. Immediately after a mission, foods and beverages that have a moderate to high GI should be consumed. During recovery and maintenance, foods with a low GI are preferred.

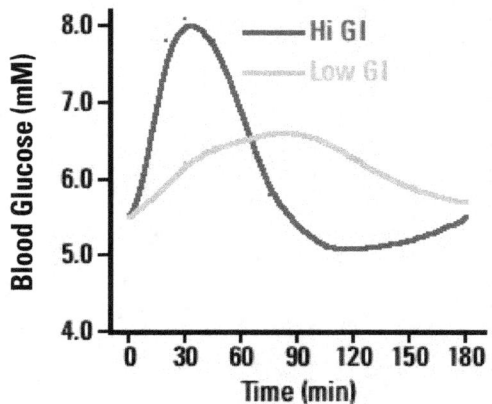

Rehydration

Fluid requirements can vary from 2–16 liters/day depending on:

- Workload.
- Level of heat stress.
- Sweat rates.

Sweat loss varies depending on age, training, and acclimation status, exercise intensity and duration, air temperature, humidity, wind velocity, cloud cover, clothing, and individual sweat rates.

The adequate fluid intake for men between 19–50 years of age is 13 cups/day. On average, 20–25% of the fluid comes from food and 75–80% from beverages. Plain water, coffee, tea, soups, fruits, and vegetables also provide fluids and support hydration. A small amount of caffeine in tea or coffee (< 200 mg) should not negatively affect hydration status, but if more caffeine is taken in, fluid balance may be negatively affected.

For each liter of sweat lost, a loss between 115–690 mg of sodium is possible in a well-conditioned warrior. If unaccustomed to working in the heat, heavy sweaters can lose as much as 2,500–5,000 mg of sodium per liter of sweat! To individualize fluid and electrolyte recommendations:

- Record weight before and after exercise to determine how much fluid should be replaced.

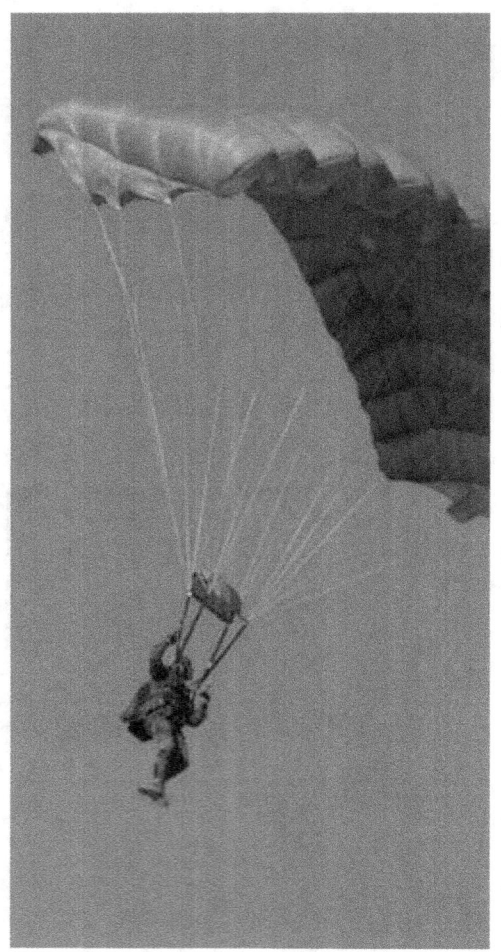

- Consume 2.5–3 cups of fluid for every pound lost.

Typically, voluntary consumption of fluids will restore only part of the fluid lost. Whenever possible, weigh yourself before and after a training so you can quantify your fluid loss. Your sweat rate during a mission will differ based on the environmental conditions, and this could intensify weight loss.

Over a period of several hours, you should ingest more water and sodium than initially lost. The total replacement volume should be between 125% and 150% of the decrease in body mass. So, if you lost 4 pounds, you would want to take in 5–6 "pounds," or 10–12 cups of water. The fluid **must** be taken in over a period of time rather than at one time. Ingesting 8–16 ounces every 20–30 minutes will allow for water absorption and minimizes water lost by urination. Do not drink more than 48 oz or 1.5 L per hour.

Fluid replacement beverages used during exercise are also appropriate for rehydration. Rehydration beverages containing a higher percentage of CHO than used during exercise are suitable, but it is better to obtain CHO from real foods. Oral Rehydration Solutions (ORS) available through the military medical supply channels can be used, but they are often higher in sodium and lower in CHO than desired.

Rehydration in the Field

A drink that will rapidly promote rehydration, is almost palatable, and contains an acceptable amount of electrolytes (although barely enough potassium) can be made in the field. The fluid is prepared by mixing ¼ strength of a fluid replacement beverage (Gatorade, Powerade, Gookinade or the like) with ¼ strength of a standard ORS. However, this drink will **not** restore glycogen because it is too low in CHO.

Sodium/Electrolyte Replacement

Sodium and potassium losses in the sweat can be quite high during prolonged physical activity, especially in warm weather. Replacing these elements is an important part of the recovery process. Most commercially available fluid replacement beverages contain electrolytes. Roughly, 1–2 grams of sodium/L of fluid (0.25 teaspoon/quart) will effectively replace the sodium lost during exercise or a mission. Also, sodium is widely present in a variety of foods and fluids, such as bagels, pretzels, tomato juice, sport drinks, and pizza.

A bit of salt will speed up rehydration more effectively than plain water. Typical commercial fluid replacement beverages contain both sodium and potassium, but recovery foods should also include foods rich in potassium. Some excellent food sources of potassium are listed to the left. You will

After a training session or mission, fluid ingestion is essential.

Drink at least two 8 oz cups of fluid every 20-30 minutes for two and a half hours after exercise.

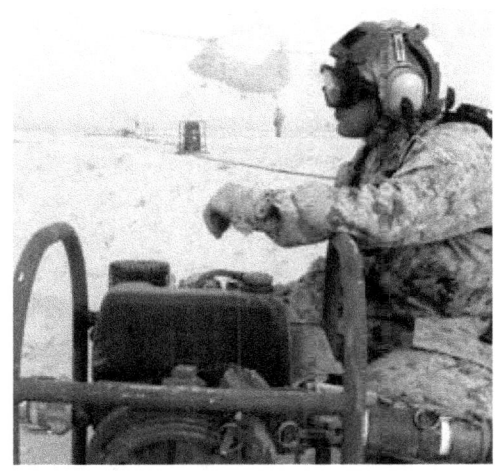

Each one quart of fluid should contain about one quarter teaspoon of salt.

Table 5–3. Good Potassium Sources	
Foods	**Beverages**
Banana	Orange juice
Apricots, dried	Tomato juice
Orange	Pineapple juice
Baked potato	Grapefruit juice
Melons	Skim milk
Yogurt	Sports drink

Note: 1 cup of orange juice or tomato juice will replace the potassium, calcium and magnesium lost in 3 quarts of sweat.

Drinking sports drinks as recreational fluids only adds calories, and artificial coloring and flavors to the diet.

notice that these foods are also good sources of CHO and most have a moderate to high GI.

Sports Drinks

Fluids providing CHO and the electrolytes, sodium and potassium, have been shown to sustain athletic performance. The genesis of sports nutrition came about when beverages were created so that CHO, electrolytes, and fluids could be consumed without having to mix, assemble or combine ingredients. The purposes of sports drinks are to:

• Maintain hydration during exercise.

• Ensure rehydration after exercise.

• Replace electrolytes lost during sweating.

• Supplement CHO stores and provide fuel for the working muscles during exercise.

• Minimize muscle from strenuous workouts.

• Protect the immune system.

Although sports drinks containing electrolytes will enhance endurance performance, many people use these drinks as a recreational fluid. This only adds calories, artificial coloring and flavors to their dietary intake. Sports drinks are recommended when exercise is longer than 60 minutes and then, only 8 oz should be ingested every 15 minutes. For activities less than one hour, water is the best choice for hydration needs. Minimal sodium and potassium are lost through sweat and glycogen stores will not be depleted during short, low intensity workouts.

General rules for fluid replacement:

• If you are sweating profusely, try to consume fluids at the rate lost (not to exceed 1.5 L/hour) or as much as tolerated if sweat rate is exceeding the rate of stomach emptying.

• Develop a plan for fluid consumption and practice it during training and operations.

• Sip frequently rather than gulp on occasion; drinking small amounts of fluids at a time are more effective than large amounts only occasionally.

• Start drinking before thirst kicks in.

The ideal CHO/electrolyte drink:

- Is not carbonated.
- Empties rapidly from the digestive tract.
- Tastes good.
- Provides energy for exercise > 1 hr.
- Delivers 9–19 grams of CHO per 8 oz.
- Contains sodium and potassium.
- Does not cause digestion problems.
- Is cool (10 to 15°C).

Sports drinks should be used during and after long bouts of exercise in hot and humid conditions. However, if real food and 100% fruit juices are available after exercise, these high CHO foods are the best electrolyte choices. Sodium is still important to take after exercise as it helps increase the desire to drink fluids and improves fluid retention.

Recovery and Commercial-Off-The-Shelf-Products (COTS)

Many Commercial-Off-The-Shelf (**COTS**) products are used for recovery. In addition, sport drinks, sports bars, gels, and other similar products are used. Some have many nutrients added, which are usually not needed or are provided in excessive amounts. The Nutrition Committee and the Dietary Supplement Committee within the Department of Defense developed criteria for various COTS categories. The criteria were prepared as guidelines on what products are safe and useful, according to scientific data, because such products are important when real food is not available. The criteria for sports bars and gels are provided below.

Sports Bars

Sports bars originated in the early 1980s when it was shown that ultramarathoners and other endurance athletes did better when provided concentrated sources of easily absorbable CHO during long training runs. Sports bars, in contrast to sport drinks, are solid, so the user must drink water to enhance digestion and absorption.

Table 5–5. Criteria for COTS Recovery Sports Bars
CHO: ≥ 53% of Energy.
CHO/PRO: ≥ 4:1.
Fiber: ≥ 1 grams.

To avoid gastrointestinal distress when fluid losses are high (> 4L), beverages should be diluted with water to half of their original strength.

Table 5–4. Suggestions for Selecting Sports Bars
Bars should **not** provide more than 100% of the DRI for vitamins and minerals.
Bars should be used with water, not sports drinks, to prevent overloading on CHO.
Bars should be high in CHO, and low in fat and protein.
Protein should not exceed 1 gram to every 4 grams of CHO.
Fat take longer to digest than CHO, so sport bars high in fat should be avoided during exercise.
High protein bars (40-30-30) should only be consumed when real food sources of protein are limited.

Table 5–5. Criteria for COTS Recovery Sports Bars
Total Fat: ≤ 30% of Energy.
Saturated Fat: ≤ 20% of Energy.
No trans fats.
Sodium: 50–240 mg.
No substances other than vitamins, minerals, protein and fat.

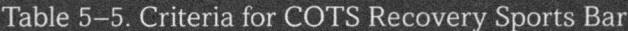

Table 5–6. COTS Recovery Sports Bars Meeting Criteria				
PRODUCTS	kcal	CHO (g)	Protein (g)	Fat (% of kcal)
Bear Valley Pemmican Mealbar	420	62	16	25
Gatorade Bar	260	46	8	17.0
Soldier Fuel (Formerly Hooah)	270	40	10	26.0
Odwalla Bars (**not** Super Protein)	240	40	6	20.8
PeakBars	244	57	4	<10
Smart Fuel MPN Oatmeal WARPBar	180	31	8	16.7
PowerBar Performance	230	45	10	10

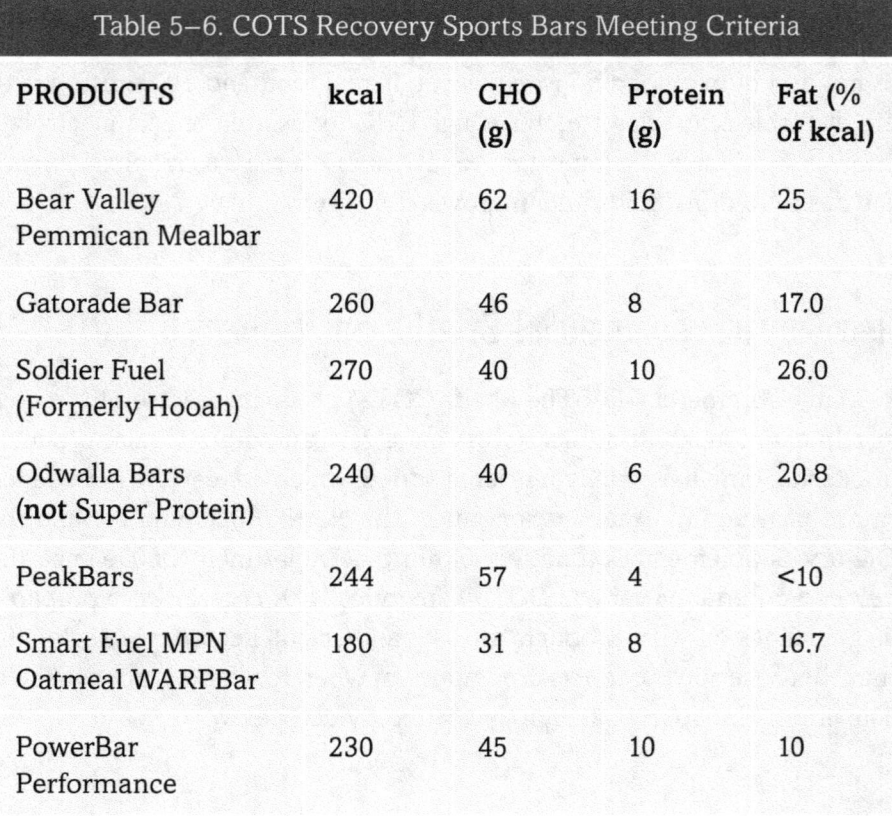

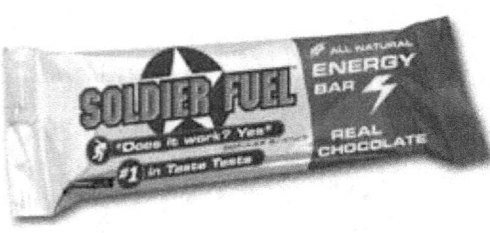

The Hooah Bar, now known as "Soldier Fuel," is an excellent recovery bar available throughout the military. It must not be mistaken for the old Hooah bar. In 2004 the manufacturer worked closely with Natick Soldier Center researchers to refine, reformulate, and improve the original bar for the military and commercial marketplace. The new bar has been rated highly by all who have tasted it. The Washington Post rated the bar above all other sports bars. The reformulated bar contains no trans fats and provides the requisite amount of CHO and protein for recovery.

Sport Gels

Sport gels were developed in the 1990s in response to complaints by endurance athletes that sports bars were difficult to digest and absorb when used during exercise. Gels have become increasingly popular for long workouts as they help maintain blood glucose and fuel the tank. However, drinking fluids is essential when using gels. Gels are popular with Warfighters because they are:

- An absorbable form of CHO, which makes eating on the go easy.

- Lightweight (1 oz) and easy to pack for many long and enduring operations lasting more than 90 minutes.

Gels may be useful after exercise for glycogen repletion when real foods are not available, but are unnecessary for short workouts, regardless of intensity.

Potential Problems with Gels

Gels are virtually 100% CHO, so it is easy to take in too much, which will lead to GI issues, such as diarrhea. Gels should be tested before combat situations to see which one works best. After over an hour of exercise, 1–2 packets are recommended, but they should be used with water, rather than sports drinks to prevent CHO overload. Listed below are the criteria for gels and various products that meet the criteria.

Table 5–7. Criteria for Commercial Off-The-Shelf Sport Gels

CHO to Protein Ratio: ≥ 4:1 ratio if any protein.

Sodium: ≤ 3 mg/g weight.

Energy: ≤ 3 kcal/g weight.

No substances other than CHO, electrolytes, protein, and caffeine.

Table 5–8. COTS Sport Gels Meeting Criteria

Products	kcal/100g	CHOg/100g	CHO:Pro ≥ 4	Sodium mg/g
Carb-BOOM!	268	66	-	1.2
Pro-Boom	170	30	-	2
Hammer Gel	253	64	-	0.6
Lava Gel	294	74	-	0.7
Clif Shot Gel	300	71	-	1.2

It is both healthier
and cheaper to
use real foods.

These CHO-rich supplements are used more often than needed because they are convenient, easy to use, and provide readily absorbable energy. Many athletes habitually eat sports foods instead of wholesome meals, even though sports products cost more than other foods. Sports drinks cost more than water, sports bars cost more than Fig Newtons, and sports gels cost more than honey.

The right combination of fluids, carbohydrates, proteins and fats in a timely manner will provide the nutritional optimization required for strenuous activities and high impact missions. The body is the vehicle that allows Warfighters to do what they have been trained to do, and it must be fed the same way as any vehicle requiring high-octane fuel. The strategies in this chapter will, in the long run, greatly benefit the mission and the Warfighter.

"Who would have thought just eating
breakfast would make the difference."

Sean Morrison, SO1, USN

6 Optimal Choices for Home Chow

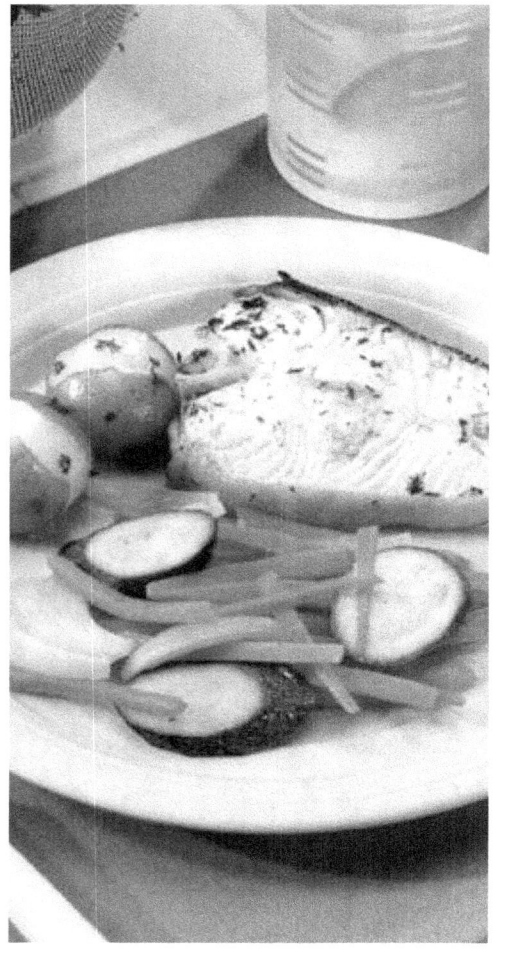

Key Points

- Foods eaten at home can impact mission performance.

- Smart shopping is the first step towards healthy meal preparation.

- Most recipes can be modified to improve nutrient composition.

- Use nutrition labels as a guide for making smart food choices.

- Every meal is important for overall health and performance.

- Aim for as many servings of fruits and vegetables as possible.

The foods and beverages consumed at home can impact mission performance. Since missions and deployments may come up suddenly, being ready to go at a moments notice is crucial. That translates into being healthy at all times! Good nutritional habits will help achieve health and better performance. This chapter provides basic information on how to eat well at home and how to avoid some of the consequences of frequently eating at fast food places.

Make the Most of Meals At Home

As families are occupied with their children's activities, taking classes in the evening, and other activities away from home, the family dinner has become an endangered activity. Only about one third of families eat dinner together each evening. Yet, children who eat seven or more meals a week with their families have fewer problems in school, are less depressed, and less likely to smoke cigarettes, drink alcohol, or use marijuana. Parents have a great opportunity and responsibility to be role models for good eating habits and provide children with nutritious meals.

Want to save money and keep off weight? Home-prepared meals are healthier and less costly than restaurant meals. According to numerous sources, home-prepared meals are higher in many nutrients (fiber, calcium, folate, iron, vitamins B6, B12, C, and E), and generally lower in saturated and trans fats. Also, less fried foods and fewer soft drinks are consumed when meals are eaten at home. All meals should be planned around the five food groups and provide foods from at least three food groups (a grain, vegetable and/or fruit, and meat and/or dairy) to ensure nutrient requirements are being met.

A balanced meal includes foods from at least 3 food groups.

Grocery Shopping

Foods prepared at home can taste good and also be healthy and nutritious. Healthy meals start with healthy ingredients. Commissaries and grocery stores offer a wide variety of foods that can be the building blocks for a healthy and nutritious meal. The key is to know which foods are the most nutritious and can best fuel the body. The list below can help guide selections while at the grocery store.

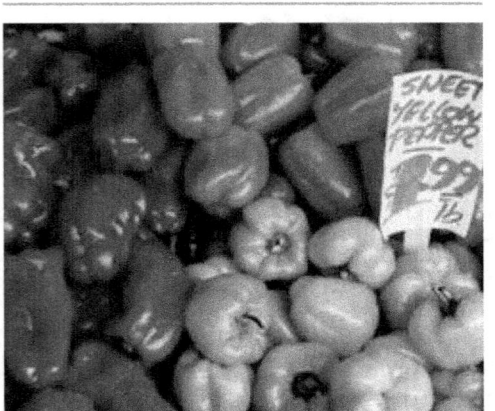

10 Tips for Grocery Shopping	
1	Plan ahead by using a shopping list.
2	Shop the perimeter of the store to include all food groups.
3	Buy a colorful array of fresh fruits and vegetables.
4	Buy whole grains with good sources of dietary fiber.
5	Buy fat-free or low-fat dairy products.
6	Buy lean protein sources.
7	Consider meat alternatives, such as beans, nuts, grains and soy products.
8	Buy heart healthy fats such as olive and canola oils.
9	Choose beverages that do not contain corn syrup and sugar.
10	Choose comfort foods with discretion by reviewing Nutrition Labels.

Recipe Modification

A number of cookbooks and online recipe sites are devoted to healthy cooking. In addition, most recipes can be modified to decrease calories, fat, sugar, and sodium, and increase fiber.

Modifying a recipe to be healthier does not have to be complicated. Some changes can be made by substituting ingredients or changing the cooking technique. Table 6–1 provides some Sensible Substitutions on how to reduce total fat, calories, sodium, and sugar, and increase fiber in recipes. The links in the left margin lead to a more extensive list of recipe modification techniques.

Table 6–1. Sensible Substitutions	
When a recipe calls for:	**Try this instead:**
Cream, 1 cup	Evaporated skim milk, 1 cup
White rice	Brown rice, bulgur, kasha, quinoa, or whole wheat couscous
Butter/margarine, ½ cup	Applesauce (or prune puree), ¼ cup + canola oil, butter or margarine, ¼ cup
Egg, 1	Egg whites, 2, or liquid egg substitute, ¼ cup
All-purpose flour, 1 cup	All-purpose flour, ½ cup + whole wheat flour, ½ cup
Pasta	Whole wheat pasta
Evaporated milk	Evaporated skim (fat-free) milk
Chocolate chips, 1 cup	Mini chocolate chips, ½ cup
Cheese, regular	Low-fat or fat-free cheese
Bacon	Lean Canadian bacon or ham
Broth	Low-sodium broth
Sour cream	Non-fat plain yogurt, 1 cup + 2 Tbsp lemon juice + 1 Tbsp skim milk
Frying in fat	Bake, broil, grill, poach, or stir fry

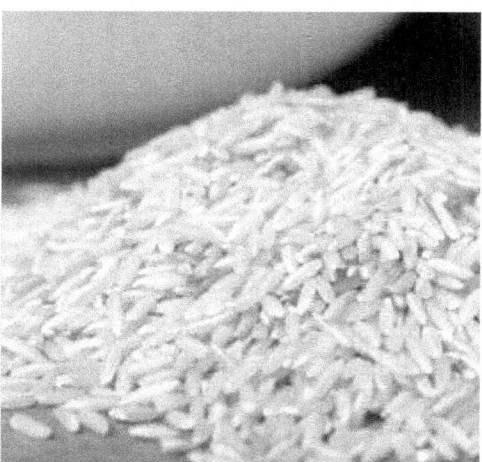

Decoding Nutrition Labels

Food labels are a valuable source of nutrition information at the grocery store. However, they can be quite intimidating if you don't know how to read them. In a recent study, researchers discovered that though most participants felt confident they understood nutritional labels and could use

Sample label for
Macaroni & Cheese.

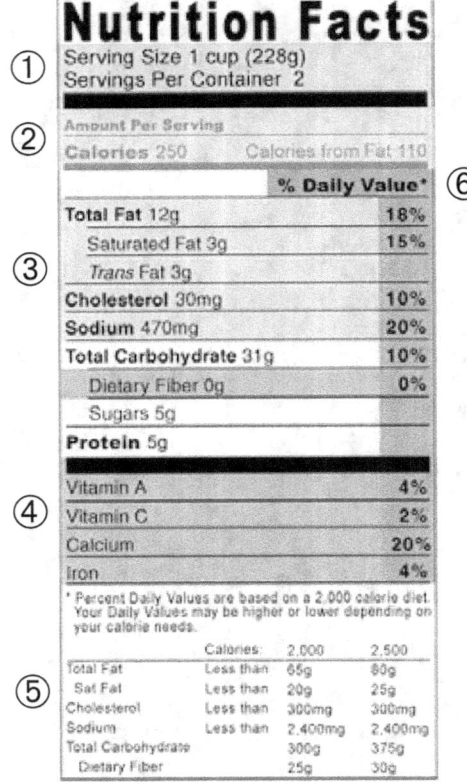

① **Start here.**

② **Check calories.**

③ **Limit these nutrients.**

④ **Get enough of these nutrients.**

⑤ **Footnote.**

⑥ **Quick guide to % DV: 5% or less is low. 20% or more is high.**

them to make healthy choices, only 37% of participants could correctly calculate the total grams of carbohydrate in a 20 oz soda.

The section below shows how to navigate around a food label to determine whether the food is a healthy choice. When shopping for groceries, the labels of food should be read and compared to determine which is healthiest.

Ingredient List

By federal regulation, any food made with more than one ingredient must carry an ingredient list on the label. The ingredients are listed in descending order according to weight, so the first ingredient is found in the largest amount.

Serving Size

The place to start when looking at the Nutrition Facts label is the serving size. It indicates a normal portion and how many servings are in the package. Always compare the label serving size with the amount that is actually eaten.

% Daily Value (DV)

Briefly discussed in Chapter 4, Percent of Daily Values appears on the label of most foods. It represents how much one serving contributes nutritionally to a 2,000-calorie-a-day diet. For example, a food is defined as "healthy" if it provides at least 10% of one or more of vitamins A or C, iron, calcium, protein, or fiber. A DV of 20% or more is considered high; try to aim high for vitamins, minerals and fiber.

Points to Consider:

• Depending on age, gender, and activity level, more or less than 2,000 kcal a day may be needed; so more or less than 100% DV may be required. Most Warfighters require at least 3,000 kcal/day, so 150% DV is needed.

• When energy requirements are unknown, the % DV offers a good reference point. If a food item lists 50% DV for cholesterol, a serving of this food provides 50% of the daily cholesterol needs for the 2,000 calorie diet.

• A DV of 5% or less is considered low; try to aim for low in total fat, saturated fat, and cholesterol.

Daily Values Footnote

This reference chart applies to healthy people requiring 2,000–2,500 calories daily, and shows daily maximum amounts for total fat, saturated fat, cholesterol, and sodium. Remember, these numbers may not be exact for you as you may require more or less calories daily.

Terminology on products is important for consumers to know and understand.

Breakfast: Off to a Healthy Start!

Forty years of breakfast-related studies have shown that jump-starting the day with breakfast is beneficial. Despite its benefits, breakfast may be the meal most often neglected or skipped. If a car can't run without fuel, how can a body? Breakfast is the body's early-morning refueling stop. After 8–12 hours without food, the body needs glucose (also known as blood sugar). A bowl of cereal with low-fat milk, toasted whole grain breads, and a piece of fresh fruit are easy, quick, and nutrient-dense selections that can be eaten at home.

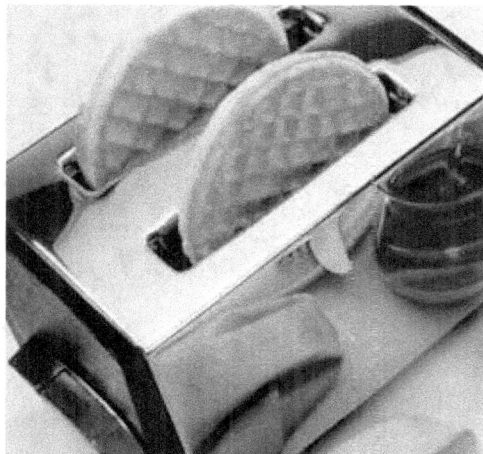

Breakfast eaters are likely to have more strength and endurance, favorable body weight, and better concentration and problem-solving ability than non-breakfast eaters.

Lunch: How to Make the Grade

A sure way to eat a nutritious lunch is by bringing it from home. Weekday brown bagging also saves you money. More importantly, you have control over what and how much is eaten and, how the food is prepared. Many non-traditional lunches can be made at home by selecting foods and beverages from the shopping tips offered in the commissary. Some useful ideas include:

- **Vegetables**: Pack them raw or lightly steamed (then chilled) with a small container of dip or salad dressing.

- **Hummus**: Use as a dip or a sandwich spread.

- **Stuffed Tomatoes or Bell Peppers**: Add tuna, chicken, egg, pasta, or rice.

- **Salads**: Don't forget salads along with sandwiches.

- **Sushi Rolls**: A terrific lunchbox fare.

- **Trail Mix**: Make a trail mix with raisins or other dried fruit combined with a whole-grain cereal or air-popped popcorn.

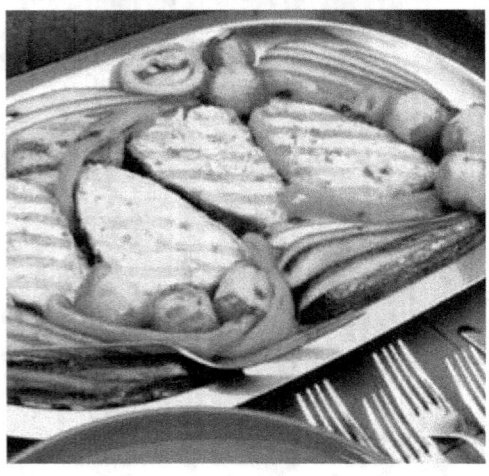

- **Fruit**: Grab several pieces of fruit to go and try some with low-fat yogurt.

Lunch is a great time to eat fruits and vegetables. Both fresh fruits and vegetables are nutrient packed, satisfying foods that will replenish glycogen, and help with hydration.

Dinner: Fueling for the Night

Dinner should not be the largest meal of the day. However, food records provided by Warfighters indicate that most calories consumed, especially during the workweek, occur in the evening hours. This is because other meals and snacks have not been consistently eaten throughout the day. Lack of time preparing for dinner and poor planning are also issues. Although planning takes time, and shopping for foods is a must, many nutritious meals can be prepared ahead of time or within 30 minutes after getting home. The following are quick dinner strategies:

- Buy pre-cooked meats to heat in the microwave.

- Use meats and fish in vacuum bags with pasta or rice.

- Use bagged lettuce, baby carrots, and spinach.

- Mix canned chili beans with diced tomatoes and precooked chicken.

- Use canned fruit in natural juices with chocolate syrup as a dessert.

- Prepare a double batch and freeze half for another meal.

Other examples of easy, yet nutritious, dinner ideas include:

- Whole grain pasta or rice with lean meat/fish and vegetables.

- Whole grain rice and beans with salsa.

- Sirloin steak, baked potato, and salad.

- Salmon, sweet potato, and vegetables.

- Pizza with Canadian bacon and vegetables.

- Caesar salad with chicken and garlic toast.

- Sandwiches made with whole grain bread, lean meat, lettuce, and tomato (grain, meat and vegetable groups).

Cooking foods, such as rice, pasta, and other grains, in large quantities can provide the staples for quick meal planning throughout the week. Adding lean meats and vegetables to the grill are other ways to end the day with a nutritious meal before bedtime.

Fruits and Vegetables—More Matters

Current evidence shows that diets rich in fruits and vegetables are associated with improved health, reduced risk of chronic diseases, and some types of cancer. Fruits and vegetables are high in fiber and water, and low in calories. The term "nutrient density" has been used several times, and another important term is "energy density." The relationship between the number of calories in a food and the weight or volume of the food is called "energy density." Although people have difficulty limiting the amount of calories they eat, most seem to be able to limit the volume, due to satiety, or the feeling of fullness. Fruits and vegetables provide good substitutes for energy-dense foods, and provide satiety with fewer calories. Eating several servings of fruits and vegetables will aid in weight management and provide the nutrients required for good health and disease prevention.

Calcium, potassium, fiber, magnesium, and vitamins A, C and E are the nutrients most lacking in the diet. Fruits and vegetables are rich in these nutrients, and half of your plate should consist of fruits and vegetables.

It is important to get as many servings of fruit and vegetables a day as possible to maximize performance and health. According to the latest research, men, on average, consume less fruit and vegetables than required for good health and cancer prevention. For instance, most men consume less than four servings of fruits and vegetables each day, despite needing almost twice that amount. Every Warfighter should consume at least 2.5 cups of fruit and 4 cups of vegetables. This is not always possible during deployments, but it is when at home. Eat at least six servings of fruits and vegetables a day and choose a variety to benefit from the different vitamins, minerals, and other nutrients each choice offers. Fruits and vegetables are the super foods that will promote health and performance, maintain weight, and provide fluid for hydration, as just a few of the benefits.

A 25-year old male exercising more than 1 hour per day needs 2.5 cups of fruit and 4 cups of vegetables every day.

Table 6–2. Reasons to Eat A Variety of Fruits and Vegetables Each Day

Packed with vitamins and minerals.

Reduces the risk of heart disease, stroke, and some cancers.

An excellent source of fiber and antioxidants.

Helps maintain a healthy weight.

Taste delicious and a variety to choose from.

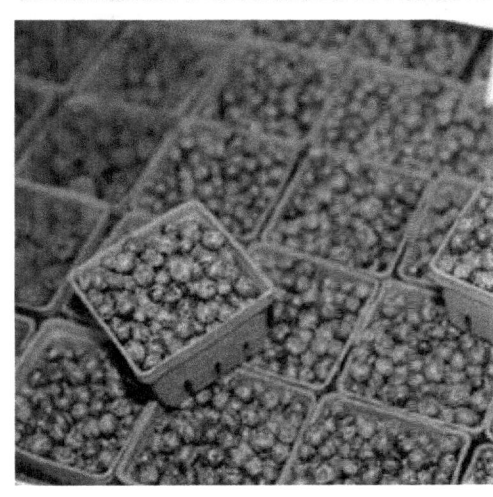

7 Optimal Choices for Eating Out

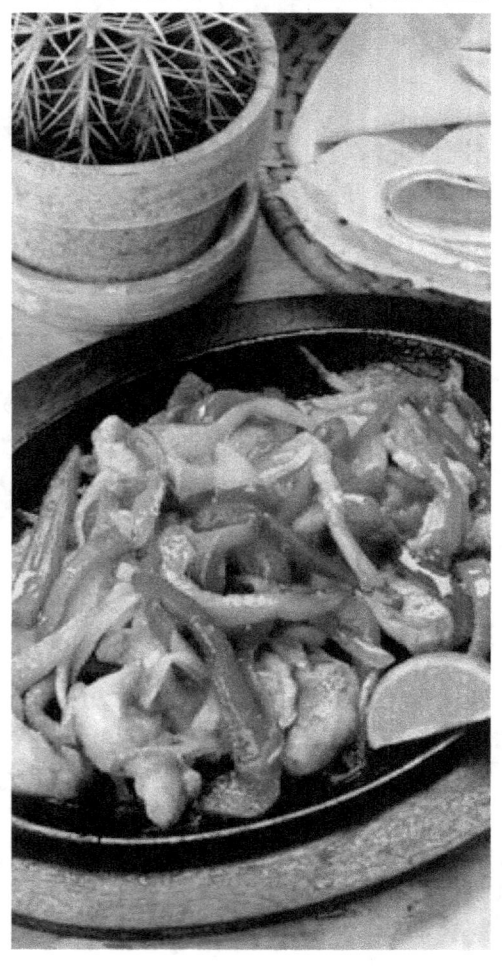

Key Points

- Not all restaurants are equal. Choose the restaurant wisely.

- Eating out can be healthy if careful meal selections are made.

- Selecting fruits and vegetables as a part of the meal adds vitamins, minerals and fiber, and helps reduce fat and calories.

- Fast food restaurants have healthy alternatives to the high-fat burger and fries. Make sensible food choices.

The trend toward eating more meals away from home reflects a growing demand for convenience, entertainment, and a variety of ethnically diverse foods. Active schedules, training requirements, and deployments make eating a majority of meals away from home appealing—it is simpler than cooking at home. Americans eat at least one-third of their calories away from home. To maximize mental agility, stamina, and health, healthy food and beverage selections are critical when eating out at fast food places, dining facilities, restaurants, social events, or when traveling. This chapter will present information on how to maintain a high-performance diet when eating away from home.

Choose Restaurants Wisely

On average, many foods prepared and eaten out tend to be less nutrient dense and have more calories than foods prepared at home. However, restaurant and fast food meals do not have to be unhealthy. By being informed and by asking appropriate questions, the guidelines of a healthy diet can be maintained and the benefits of eating out can be enjoyed. The good news is that when you don't want to cook, are too busy, or just want to enjoy a dining out experience, it is possible to eat healthy. Some suggestions on how to choose a restaurant include:

- Plan ahead: Select a restaurant where food is cooked to order rather than where the food is made ahead of time.

- Avoid places with dessert carts and all-you-can-eat or buffet-only specials.

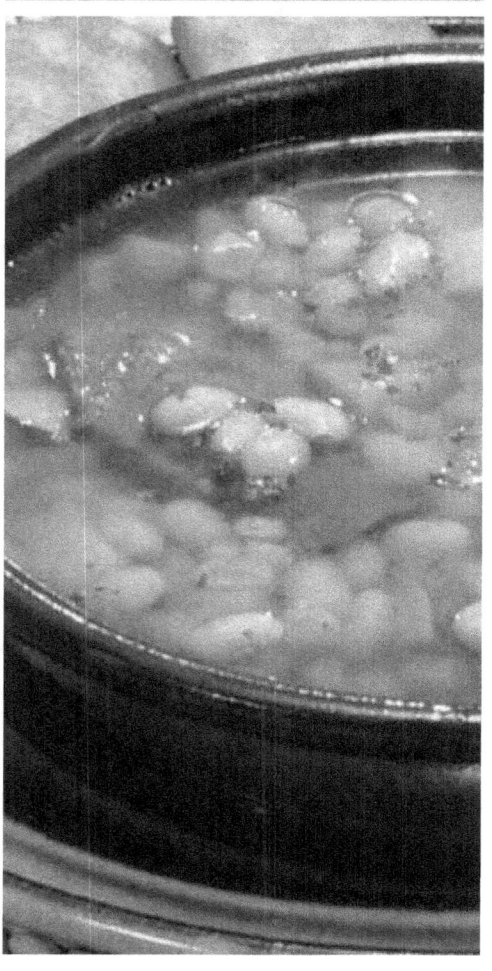

- Try Greek restaurants that serve Mediterranean-type meals.

- Choose healthy ethnic foods from Chinese, Japanese, Thai, Indian, Italian, French, and Middle Eastern eateries.

- Skip the hot dogs and pizza and search for fast food places that offer healthy options such as fruit, yogurt, soup, sushi, salads, sandwiches, or wraps.

- Look for a place that offers menus with nutrition information.

- Find a place to eat before you're starving or you will tend to choose quickly. Plan ahead and give yourself time to choose. If you are very hungry, buy an apple or other healthy snack to tide you over.

Choosing a Nutritious Meal

Once at your restaurant of choice, read the menu carefully to select a high carbohydrate, nutrient dense meal. The following menu strategies are usually available in most restaurants. Select a hearty meal that fits into your nutrition plan. The following guidance will assist with meal selections.

Appetizers

Appetizers are tasty but they cause mindless nibbling, which adds fat and calories. If you're starving, have the bread but skip the butter. Have the waiter remove the bowl of chips or peanuts, or the basket of bread, after you've had a small portion. Select an appetizer that is neither fried nor covered with cheese.

Soups can be a great appetizer or entrée.

Many soups are low in calories and will help fill you up and satisfy your hunger. Select a broth or other light soup, such as a vegetable soup. Avoid cream soups which are high in fat.

Salads are more than just rabbit food.

Fresh vegetable salads are great, but ask for a balsamic vinaigrette, a fat-free, or a reduced-calorie salad dressing on the side to control how much or how little you add.

If a salad bar is included in the meal, avoid cheese, croutons, fried or crispy meat, bacon bits, potato and Caesar salads, creamed pastas, and coleslaw. In other words, keep it simple. Fill the plate with lettuce, spinach, other greens, and all the colorful vegetables. Add juicy red tomatoes, bright orange shaved carrots, green peas, yellow and red bell peppers, dark green broccoli, white cauliflower, crispy cucumbers, and other vegetables to turn your greens into a fiesta of colors.

Main Meal

The main course, or main meal, can be a healthy affair.

- Choose entrees with fruits and vegetables as key ingredients. Enjoy the flavors they offer. Fruits and vegetables are a good source of dietary fiber, as well as a source of many vitamins and minerals. Or, order a side of fresh, steamed veggies and make it a meal.

- If you want to eat less, order two appetizers, or an appetizer and a salad, or soup and ½ sandwich as your meal. Ensure you are ordering the low-fat options. Or, if portions at the restaurant are large, split one meal with your dinner partner.

Meat/Fish

A reasonable portion of steak or other meat is 3–6 oz. Meat portions should be about the size of a deck of cards, not the size of your plate. Pass on gravies or heavy sauces, which add a significant amount of fat. Season your meat with pepper, chunky salsa, or herbs.

- Chicken can be great if it is not fried or consumed with its skin.

- Pork, "the other white meat," is good, but can be fatty. Skip the ribs and go for a ham steak instead.

- Select healthy food preparations. Ask that the meat or fish be steamed, poached, broiled, baked, grilled, or roasted instead of deep-fried or prepared in butter or oil.

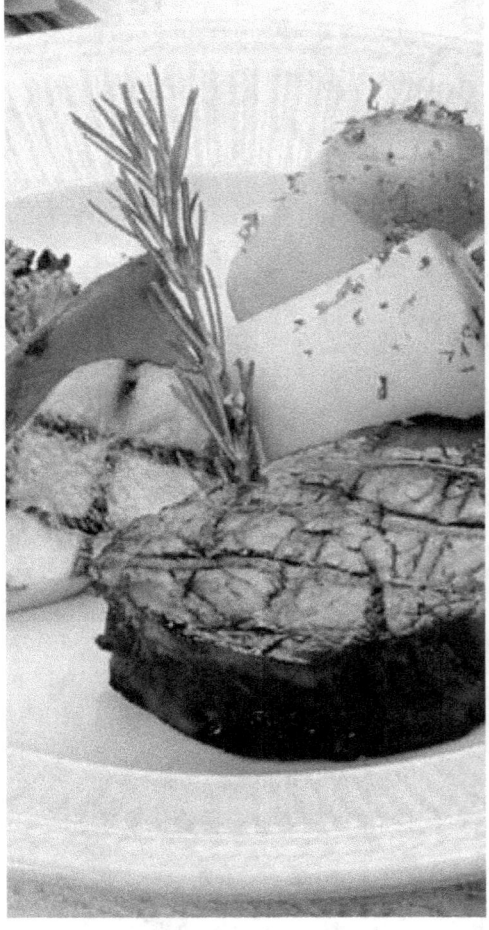

Starches/Carbohydrates

Several tips for ordering carbohydrates:

- Order a baked potato (without the sour cream and butter) or plain rice—not fried rice. Avoid onion rings, other fried vegetables and au gratin or Delmonico potatoes.

- Order pasta with marinara (tomato-based sauce), not cream sauce.

- Ask for salsa or chives with a baked potato instead of high-fat sour cream, butter, cheese, or bacon. They are very low in calories and a healthy alternative with a lot of flavor.

- Choose whole-grain bread and dishes made with brown rice.

- Beans, while usually a good choice, may have been prepared with unhealthy lard. Ask your server how they are prepared.

Vegetables

Order two servings of steamed vegetables when possible. Stay away from cheesy and battered, deep-fried vegetables or those prepared in oil or butter. Grilled vegetables are a great option.

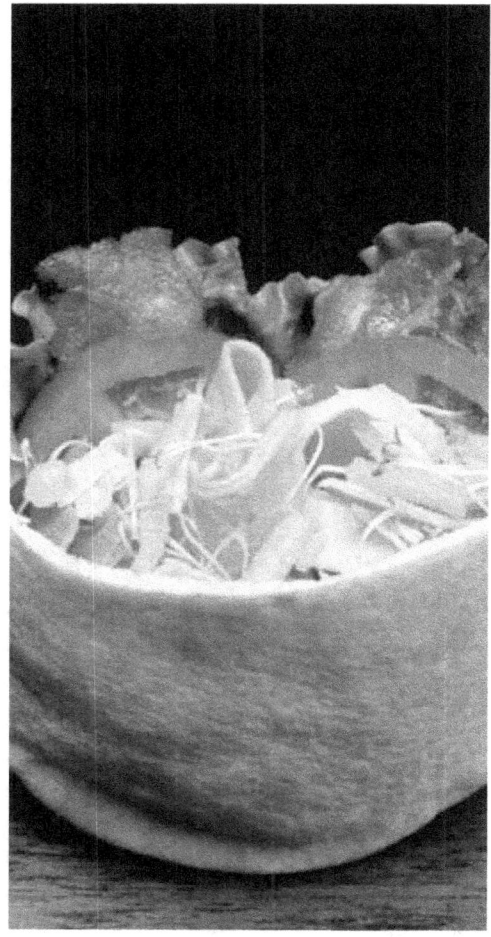

Other Main Courses

Casseroles

Casseroles are tasty but can be very high in fat and calories. Avoid casseroles and foods with heavy cream or cheese sauces. Pot pies are primarily high-fat gravy with little meat or vegetables.

Pastas

When ordering pasta dishes, look for tomato-based sauces (marinara) rather than cream-based sauces. Tomato-based sauces are much lower in fat and calories. In addition, the tomato sauce can count as a vegetable: a win-win situation. To help fill you up, order an extra serving of steamed vegetables to mix with your pasta. If you add meat, select grilled chicken or salmon instead of the sausage. Add a small amount of grated Parmesan cheese for additional flavor.

Sandwiches

Sometimes you aren't hungry or don't have time for a long sit-down meal. In that case, a sandwich is a great alternative. Here are some helpful tips about ordering a healthy sandwich:

- Select sandwiches on whole wheat, pita, multi-grain breads. Choose low-fat deli meats and cheeses, mustard, relish, ketchup, or low-fat mayonnaise. Add flavor and vitamins with roasted sweet peppers, lettuce tomato, jalapenos, and chopped olives (small amount).

- Order sandwiches with mustard rather than mayonnaise or "special sauce." Mustard adds zing with virtually no calories.

Beverages

It is important to stay adequately hydrated, but an easy way to gain weight is by drinking sodas, alcohol, and milk, which only add unnecessary, empty calories. With or in between meals, select water, diluted fruit juice, skim or low-fat milk, or unsweetened tea or coffee. Energy drinks, CHO-electrolyte beverages, sweetened tea, and juice drinks can promote weight gain.

If wine is desired, have one glass with the main dish. Drink water with a wedge of lemon while waiting for the main entree.

Drink only one glass of wine very slowly. Take time to enjoy the taste by sipping it slowly rather than just consuming it.

Dessert

Try an herbal tea or decaffeinated coffee. If you can't resist dessert, order sorbet, fresh berries or fruit, sorbet, frozen yogurt, or ice milk. Angel food cake with strawberries, plain Jell-O, or poached fruit is a refreshing dessert. If you want something outrageous, split it with your dining partner or eat half only.

Share a dessert with a friend.
Half the dessert equals half the calories.

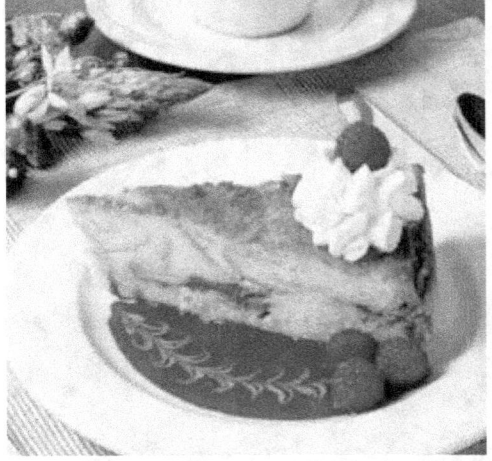

Other Helpful Tips:

- Stop eating when you are full—your body gives you satiety clues.

- Eat slowly and take time to taste and savor the food. Enjoy your dinner conversation.

- Remember not to deprive yourself of foods you love. All foods can fit into a well-balanced diet. Small portions are the key.

- Ask how an appealing dish is prepared and request healthy substitutions (baked instead of fried, olive oil instead of butter).

- Ask for a "doggie bag" up front and set aside half of your meal prior to eating. This will help ensure that you will not overeat. You will have another meal of your leftovers the next day.

- Try to avoid dishes described as au gratin, buttered, buttery, creamed, crispy, escalloped, fried, hash, hollandaise, in cheese sauce, in cream sauce, in gravy, pan-fried, pot pie, rich, sautéed, stewed, and with bacon or sausage.

Fruit and Vegetables When Eating Out

Remember, when it comes to fruit and vegetables, **more matters**. Order these items when eating out:

- Select 100% fruit or vegetable juices for breakfast, lunch, dinner, or a snack.

- Order a fruit cup for breakfast to get a good day's start.

- Make a lunch meal out of vegetable soup and a side salad.

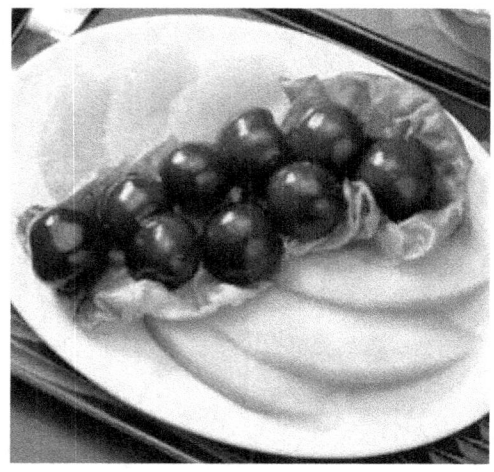

- Order sandwiches or wraps that include vegetables, such as lettuce, tomato, sprouts, green pepper, cucumber, or other raw vegetables.
- Select an apple, orange, or banana—perfect fast food when on the run.

Table 7–1. Do's and Don'ts of Ordering When Eating Out	
Do's	**Don'ts**
100% fruit juice.	Juice (many juices have corn syrup).
Fresh fruit or fresh fruit cup.	Fruit in syrup.
Steamed vegetables.	Fried vegetables or cooked in butter.
Wraps and burritos without mayo.	Hoagie or sub roll with mayo.
Extra vegetables or any vegetable combination.	French fries, fried vegetables, salads with lots of creamy dressing.
Vegetable pizza (with > 3 veggies).	"Meat lover's" pizza.
Baked potato or sweet potato.	French fries or potato salad.
Salad bar.	Skip the lettuce and go straight for the mayonnaise pastas.
Fresh fruit with low-fat whipped cream.	Tarts, cheese cake, Danishes, and other pastries.

Fast Foods

Fast foods are a way of life!

Selecting fast food items that will meet your nutrient requirements and match your activity patterns and performance demands is possible at fast food restaurants. Fast foods can provide the protein, carbohydrate, and adequate vitamins and minerals, but it takes careful planning. The carbohydrate, protein, and fat (CPF) distribution of typical fast food meals is illustrated. Often 40%–60% of the calories are from fat. Also, most menu items are very high in sodium, which can contribute to high blood pressure, and dietary fiber is usually lacking or quite low. Americans consume about half the recommended daily amount of fiber.

Suggestions for Choosing Fast Foods

- Look for meals that provide 800–900 calories, have < 30 grams of fat and < 1,000 milligrams of sodium.

- Select regular size portions and avoid jumbo-, giant-, deluxe-, and super-sized options.

- Balance a fast food meal with the rest of the day's dietary intake.

- Order a single burger without special toppings and sauces.

- Avoid chicken and fish that are breaded and fried.

- Select cheese or vegetarian pizzas. Avoid extra cheese, pepperoni and sausage since they contribute additional fat.

Table 7–2. Substitutions at Fast Food Restaurants		
Skip This	**Try Instead**	**Calories Saved**
Double cheeseburger	Cheeseburger	280
Super fries	Small fries	330
Burrito supreme	Soft chicken taco	209
Stuffed potato	Baked potato, plain	348
Pepperoni lovers pizza	Cheese pizza, 2 slices	174
Large regular soda	Spritzer water	310
Breaded chicken sandwich	Grilled chicken	205

Fast Foods and the Web

Many fast-food restaurants have their menus on the web—here are a few to check out.

- Taco Bell:
  http://www.yum.com/nutrition/menu.asp

- Kentucky Fried Chicken:
  http://www.kfc.com/nutrition/zerotransfat.asp

- McDonalds:
  http://www.mcdonalds.com/usa/eat/nutrition_info.html

- Pizza Hut:
  http://www.pizzahut.com/Nutrition.aspx

- Subway:
  http://www.subway.com/subwayroot/MenuNutrition/index.aspx

- Dunkin Donuts:
  http://www.dunkindonuts.com/aboutus/nutrition/

- Starbucks:
  http://www.starbucks.com/retail/nutrition_info.asp

- Arby's:
  http://www.arbys.com/nutrition/

- Chick-Fil-A:
  http://www.chick-fil-a.com/Nutrition.asp

- Domino's:
  www.dominos.com/PublicEN/Site+Content/Primary/See+the+Menu

- Wendy's:
  http://www.wendys.com/food/NutritionLanding.jsp

- Burger King:
  http://www.bk.com/#menu=3,-1,-1

- Five Guys:
  http://www.fiveguys.com/menu.html

- Popeyes:
  http://www.popeyes.com/nutrition/pop_nutrition.pdf

8 Healthy Snacking

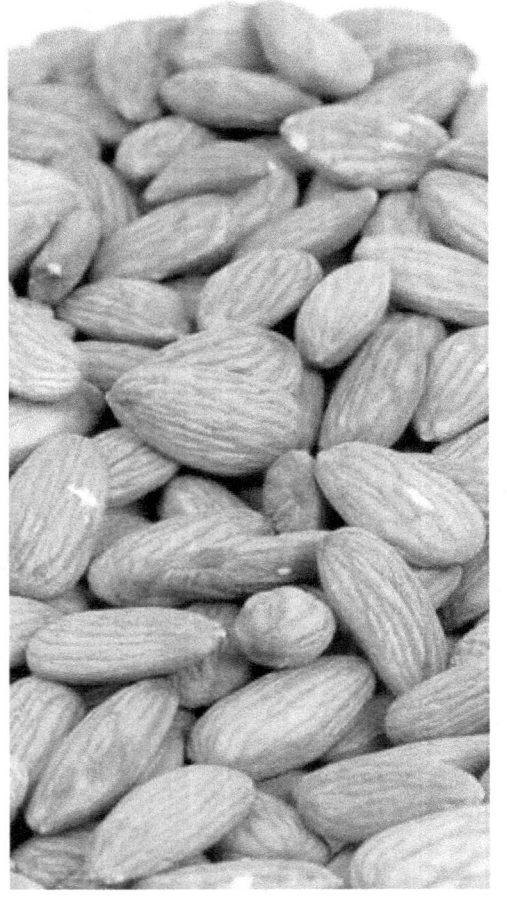

Key Points

- Snacking, or "eating between regular meals," is important to help maximize performance and maintain mental and physical acumen.

- Healthy snacks can help increase energy and alertness without promoting weight gain.

- Keep nutrient dense snacks at home, work, or "on the go."

- Snacks for night operations should include foods low in carbohydrate and high in protein.

- Snacks high in water, such as fruit, are great for warm weather operations.

- Snacks high in carbohydrate are good to consume when exercising in the cold.

- Avoid high-fat snacks during missions.

Energy expenditure can be extremely high on given days and during various operations, and it is often difficult to eat enough at meals. Snacking becomes very important during these times and may help maintain performance and mental acuity. In addition, most of us snack at various times during the day and evening anyway, so it becomes important to look at what constitutes healthy snacks.

Healthy Snacking and Making the Most of Snacks

Most people think snacking is unhealthy and leads to weight gain. That notion, however, has emerged because most people don't eat healthy snacks. If you don't care about gaining weight, just about any snack will do; but if you want to maintain weight and perform well, then your selection of snacks is critical.

Carefully chosen, snacks can fill nutritional gaps and boost energy without causing weight gain. Think through a typical day. How often and where do you usually snack? Are the snacks you choose high in nutrients or load-

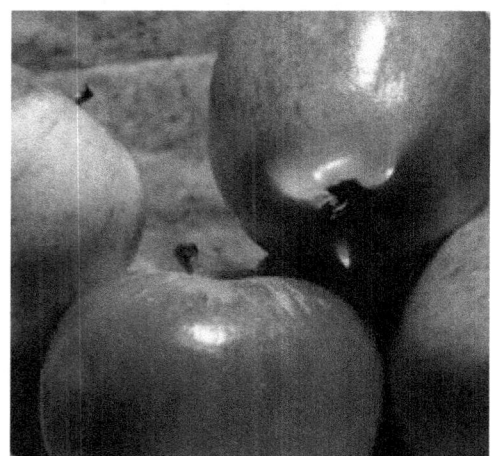

ed with "empty" calories? If you aren't sure, some tips to help promote healthy snacking follow.

Snacking Tips

- Plan snacks ahead of time.
- To stave off hunger longer, pick snacks with protein and a heart-healthy fat.
- Match snacks to activity level.
- Choose fresh fruit for a sweet snack rather than candy or cookies.
- Be conscious of portion sizes.
- If possible, do not snack in front of the TV or computer it is too easy to overeat.
- Avoid all-day nibbling.
- Choose a snack that provides dietary fiber as well as other nutrients (unless the snack is for a mission).

The Snacking Environment

Satisfy the "snack tooth" urge with these convenient and healthy choices.

Home

Stock the fridge and freezer with:

- Low-fat varieties of yogurt, cottage cheese, cheese, milk and frozen yogurt.
- Lean deli meats.
- Whole fruits and cut-up raw veggies.
- 100% fruit and vegetable juices, and frozen juice bars.

Stock up on microwave snacks:

- Single serving soups.
- Whole wheat pita bread or English muffins with tomato sauce, Italian herbs and low-fat cheese for instant pizza.
- Fat-free refried beans and/or salsa with whole wheat tortillas or baked chips.
- Low-fat cheddar cheese and a leftover baked potato or plain sweet potato.

Work

Stash snacks at work

Good snacks should be kept at work in case of late or long work days or when are unable to pack a snack from home. Things to keep at work may include:

- Vegetable or bean soups in heat-and-serve cans or instant dry soup cups.
- Snack-size cereal boxes; instant oatmeal packets; boxes of raisins or other dried fruit, or whole-grain pretzels.
- Mini cans or pouches of water-packed tuna or chicken.
- A jar of natural peanut or almond butter with whole grain crackers or rice cakes.
- Beef jerky.
- Single-serve fruit cups packed in light syrup or water.
- Dry roasted, unsalted nuts.
- Low-fat granola bars.
- Canned or boxed 100% fruit juice.
- Packages of low-fat microwave popping popcorn.
- Graham crackers.
- Raisin-nut mixes.

Find vending machines with food-group snacks:

- Peanuts, raisins, trail mix.
- Low-fat granola bars.
- Whole fruit.
- 100% fruit juice.
- Low-fat milk or yogurt.
- Pretzels.

When your duty section has the proverbial "snack station:"

If there is a snack station, talk with the POC to see if they can stock some healthier items. Suggest the following items to include in the snack station:

- Baked chips.
- Beef jerky.
- Dried fruit or fruit cups packed in water or light syrup.

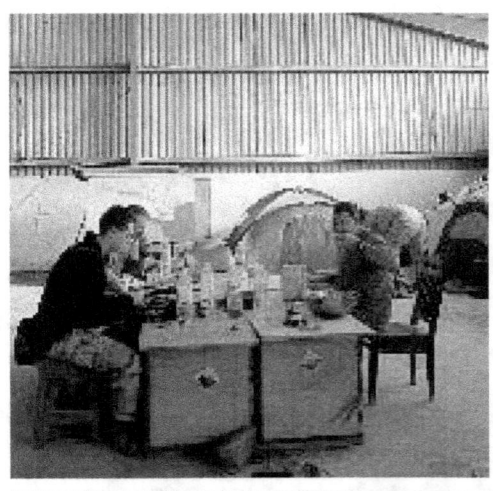

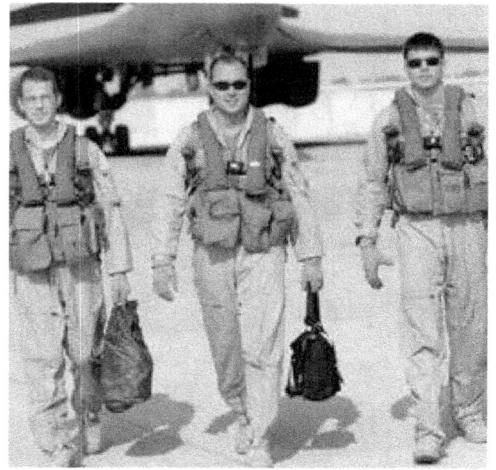

Table 8–1. Possible Night Time Snacks for Ops

Power Bars/Peanut Toffee/Cool Mint Chocolate Clif Bar

Bagel with Cream Cheese

Crackers with Hardboiled Egg

Protein/CHO Beverage

Trail Mix

Crackers with Peanut Butter or Cheese

Dark Chocolate (semi-sweet)

Hot Tea or Iced Tea

Coffee

Coffee Flavored Yogurt

- Mini cans or pouches of tuna packed in water.
- Frozen fruit bars.
- Low-fat yogurt.
- High-fiber cereal or low-fat granola bars.
- Individual snack packs of vegetables or fruit with dip.
- Instant oatmeal packets.
- Roasted, unsalted nuts.

"On the Go"

Choose wisely at convenience stores or malls where the temptation of high-calorie, high-fat options abound. Choose:

- Bagged pretzels.
- Whole grain bagels with peanut butter or light cream cheese.
- Frozen yogurt or small fruit smoothies (made with real fruit).
- 100% fruit juice.
- Beef jerky.
- Baked chips.
- Snack size package of unsalted nuts.

What Foods/Snacks are Best for Different Occasions?

Operations at Night

Foods low in CHO and high in protein are appropriate for night operations. Avoid foods high in the amino acid "tryptophan," which is known to "promote" sleep. Choose:

- CHO made with whole grains such as sports bars, bagels, tortilla wraps, and pita bread.
- Add protein-rich foods to CHO, like low-fat cream cheese, or mashed canned beans like hummus, refried pinto or black beans.
- Protein/CHO beverages described in the fluids section of Chapter 3.
- Caffeine-rich foods, yogurts with coffee flavor, caffeine chewing gum, dark chocolate, and beverages such as coffee and tea.

Caffeine always needs to be mentioned, even in the snack food section, while on the topic of "staying awake." Products that contain caffeine, however, especially manufactured foods, are not required to have the caffeine dosage reported on the food label. Therefore, it is possible to overdose on caffeine while being unaware of how much has been consumed. For most, between 200–400 mg of caffeine/day, or 2–3 cups of coffee, is adequate as a stimulant and should not pose any serious side effects.

Caffeine is less effective for a person who routinely drinks (much) coffee or caffeinated beverages, but it will work as a stimulant if consumed infrequently.

Sleep-Enhancing Foods

Foods appropriate for promoting sleep should be high in CHO and contain a small amount of protein. As mentioned above, foods with tryptophan are great "sedative/sleep-enhancing snooze foods." Table 2 provides a list of foods high in tryptophan: such foods should be eaten when you are trying to go to sleep, and conversely, avoided on night operations. The foods with the most tryptophan are listed first.

Operations in the Heat

Conducting missions in warm to hot environments require foods that provide fluid. Fluid replacement beverages are most useful, but when fruit is available, the fluid and nutrients contained in these foods are excellent. Foods that require fluids for digestion and those that naturally promote thirst, such as foods high in fat or salt, should be minimized.

Table 8–2. Foods Containing Tryptophan–Not Suitable for Night Operations*	
Oats	Bananas
Fish (Tuna, Halibut, Sardines, Salmon)	Poultry (Chicken, Turkey)
Dried Dates	Sesame
Milk, Yogurt	Chickpeas
Tofu	Sunflower Seeds
Cottage Cheese, Mozzarella Cheese	Pumpkin seeds
Red Meat (Hamburger, Steak)	Peanuts
Eggs	Ham

*Remember: try to also avoid combinations of these foods (such as pizza and ham)!

Table 8–3. Snacks to Eat During Operations in the Heat	
Watermelon	Oranges
Strawberries	Fruit Popsicles
Grapes	CHO Beverages with Electrolytes

Operations in the Cold

Operations in cold weather require foods that produce heat. Foods high in CHO produce more heat during digestion than either fat or protein. Drinking hot beverages, such as cocoa, coffee, and teas, increases body temperature, enhances mental awareness, and provides comfort. Table 8–4 provides suggestions for snacks to eat when the weather is cold.

Table 8–4. Snacks to Eat During Cold Weather Operations	
Granola/Power Bars	Fig Newtons

Table 8–4. Snacks to Eat During Cold Weather Operations	
Hot Chocolate	Bagel with Jam
Pretzels	Popcorn, Corn Chips or Tortilla Chips
Trail Mix	Crackers (any kind)

Healthful snacks for the chip-and-dip crowd.

Sustained Operations

By definition, **sustained operations** are those missions or training sessions where work is continuous for over 24 hours with minimal sleep, and few rest periods. During these times it is important to receive adequate amounts of CHO as well as fluid. The specific types of snacks will depend on the environment and how long the work must be sustained. In general, high-fat foods should be avoided and CHO with some protein should be eaten. A combination of the recommendations already made would be best, depending on the environmental conditions.

Table 8–5. Snacks to Eat During Sustained Operations	
Granola/Power Bars	Oatmeal Cookies
Hot or Cold Protein/CHO Beverage	Bagel with Jam
Pretzels	Trail Mix
Dried or Fresh Fruit	Crackers with Hard Cheese

Occasional Snacking and Discretionary Calories

There comes a time when being healthy is not a goal. Discretionary calories in snacks are calories used to satisfy hunger and personal food cravings. The amount of these snacks will depend upon whether weight maintenance, gain, or loss, is desired. Regardless, it is still wise to be selective, so if a candy bar or other sweets is essential to well-being, choose one as high in CHO and as low in fat as possible: peppermint patties, MARS Chocolate Chip Whole Grain Bar, 3 Musketeers, or gum drops, for example. Remember, these foods are not encouraged because they provide **only** energy—no vitamins or minerals, which are essential to process the energy. However, an occasional one will certainly not hurt.

9 Secrets to Keeping Lean as a Fighting Machine

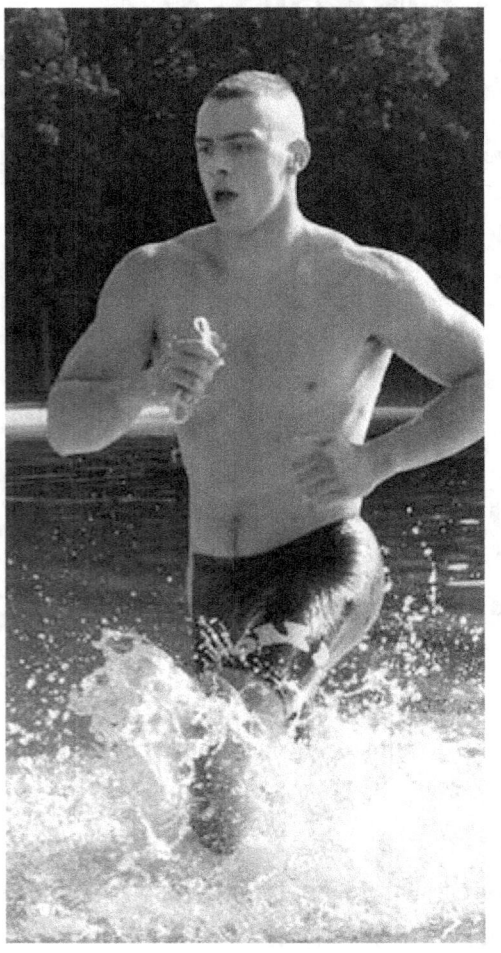

Key Points

- Consumption of carbohydrate (CHO) in defined amounts is the most important fuel strategy for all forms of exercise.

- Depletion of glycogen stores will result in poor performance in the weight room and endurance training sessions, such as a pack run.

- Improper nutrient intake and low muscle glycogen stores may increase the risk of musculoskeletal injuries.

- CHO ingestion improves the use of amino acids when they are ingested together.

- Drinking too much plain water can pose performance pitfalls during prolonged missions/exercise sessions that involve constant movement.

- Individual food preferences should be determined to avoid gastrointestinal distress during training and operations.

Warfighters must be in excellent physical condition to endure arduous physical tasks for extended periods. Endurance capacity can be greatly improved by regular physical conditioning, but it is maintained by sound nutritional practices. This chapter will discuss key dietary nuances to delay fatigue and reduce the risk of injury during and after training and/or missions. A well-fueled machine will work to its full capability and capacity; one that is inadequately fueled will not.

Fueling the Machine

Prolonged running, swimming, load carrying and/or multiple short bouts of high intensity activity, imposes significant demands on energy stores. The primary source of energy for sustained (and resistance) exercise is carbohydrate (CHO); without adequate CHO, performance goals cannot be achieved. Failure to consume enough CHO may result in:

- Fatigue.

- Poor performance.
- Irritability.
- Poor sleep patterns.
- Musculoskeletal injuries.

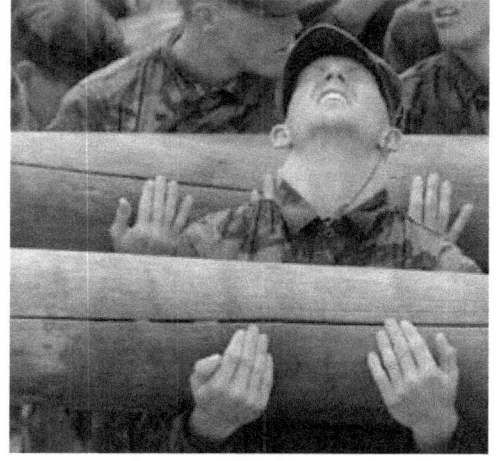

Glycogen is composed of many glucose molecules linked together.

Glycogen (our storage form of CHO) in liver and muscle is the primary source of glucose/energy for muscles (and brain) during prolonged activities. To optimize endurance performance, muscle and liver glycogen stores must be maintained. The ability to sustain performance will decrease markedly when glycogen stores are depleted: Exhaustion is certain when this happens.

Carbohydrates and the Fighting Machine

Optimizing glycogen stores is a special challenge for military personnel under sustained operations, be it during training or a mission. The most practical strategy, whenever possible, is to eat small high CHO meals frequently; this also avoids the possible discomfort of large meals. A small meal is particularly important in the morning, when liver stores may be low from not having eaten for several hours. Breaking the fast (breakfast) with a good source of CHO is critical to maintaining blood glucose and liver and muscle glycogen stores.

CHO is the most important energy-providing nutrient for endurance training.

The timing and frequency of CHO intake at various times of the day and training are crucial determinants for optimizing glycogen stores. The process is cyclical: CHO should be ingested immediately after exercise to promote muscle and liver glycogen repletion, at various times before exercise (breakfast), and at multiple intervals throughout the day. Frequent CHO ingestion will ensure a readily available source of fuel as glycogen stores become depleted.

CHO and Endurance

The figure below illustrates patterns of muscle glycogen depletion over three days, when exercising two hours per day. Subjects on a low CHO diet gradually depleted their glycogen stores over the three-day period, whereas glycogen stores were repleted between training sessions on a high CHO diet. The need to consume foods high in CHO is clear.

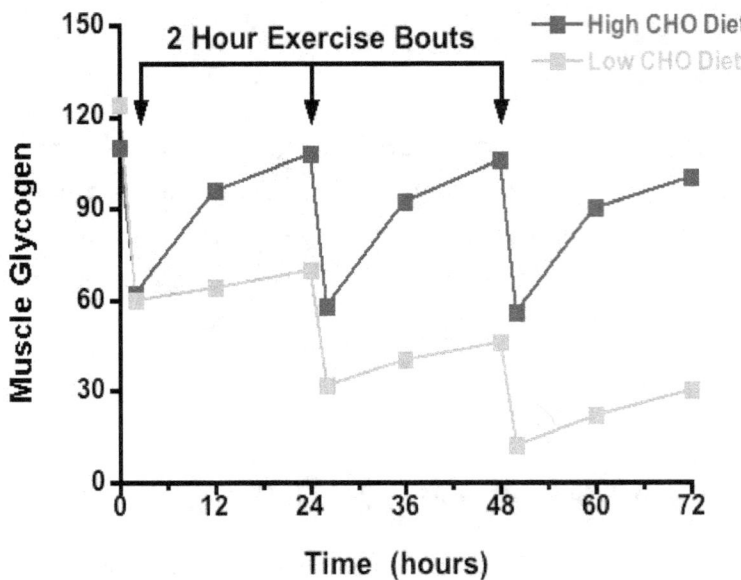

Eat 2.5–6 grams CHO per pound of body weight daily, depending on the duration of the training session.

Table 9–1. Ranges of CHO Intake for Varying Duration of Endurance Training Sessions

Exercise Time (hrs/day)	Carbohydrate (g/lb body weight)
1	2.5–4
2	3–4
3	4–5
4	4–6

Example:

Weight = 175 lbs and training is one hour each day.

2.5 x 175 kg = 437 grams of CHO

4 x 175 kg = 650 grams of CHO

CHO needs are between 437 and 650 grams per day.

Another way to think about CHO needs is in terms of energy intake. Typically, 50–70% of daily energy intake should come from CHO, and at a minimum, 400 grams of CHO should be consumed each day to ensure adequate glycogen stores. A diet providing 55% of the daily energy intake needed will almost always provide 400 grams of CHO. When energy intake is greater than 4,000 kcals, energy needs should be met by increasing fat intake. Recommendations for approximate gram amounts of CHO, protein, and fat for various energy levels are presented in Table 9–2.

CHO intake over 24 hours will typically not exceed 650 grams.

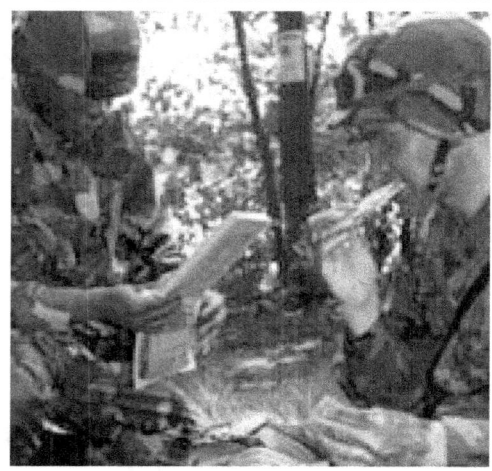

Table 9–2. Approximate Number of Grams of CHO, Protein and Fat for Various Energy Intake Levels During Sustained High-Tempo Operations			
Energy Level (kcal)	**CHO (g)**	**Protein (g)**	**Fat (g)**
3,000	450	120	80
3,500	525	135	100
4000	600	150	110
4500	625	165	150
5000	650	180	190

Because each gram of CHO provides 4 kcal, the number of grams of CHO needed can be easily calculated from energy intake. A list of various high CHO foods and the grams of CHO provided by each food is provided in Chapter 5. Complex CHO foods are preferred since they also provide vitamins and minerals in addition to CHO (see Chapter 4). Other important recommendations include:

Eat high CHO snacks *between* training sessions to replenish glycogen stores.

Consume at least 50 grams of CHO with 10–12 grams of protein immediately *after* completing a training session.

Fluid replacement beverages and a sports bar are great during recovery from long training sessions because they supply CHO, water, protein, electrolytes, vitamins and minerals.

Keep a log of all CHO foods eaten for several days to determine if CHO intake is high enough.

Protein Needs

Although protein requirements are higher for endurance training than a sedentary lifestyle, rarely is military personnel lacking in protein. Most diets provide far more than what is needed.

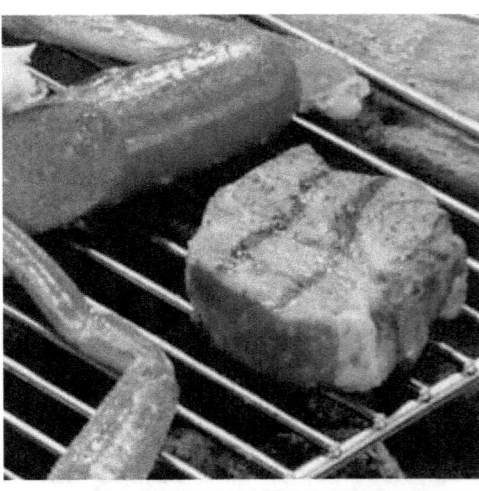

Maintaining a positive energy balance is more important than increasing protein intake for both endurance and resistance exercise training.

Importantly, if protein intake is high, and eaten at the expense of CHO, glycogen stores may be reduced and performance compromised. Protein requirements were calculated in Chapter 3 so refer to that chapter for more information. However, in general:

Protein intakes should range from
0.6–0.9 grams per lb body weight/day.

A number of factors will determine the response of the body to the ingestion of protein. These include:

- Composition of the ingested protein.

- Metabolic state: exercise or rest.

- Presence of other nutrients.

- Timing of ingestion relative to exercise.

- Interactions among all the factors above.

It is well accepted that the composition of the ingested protein is more important than the quantity. For example, amino acids (protein) from animal proteins (e.g., milk) may be superior to plant proteins. After resistance exercise skeletal muscles take up amino acids from milk proteins (such as whey and casein) faster than from soy protein. Also, during the resting state, casein protein appears to produce a stronger "anabolic" environment than whey protein. This is because the amino acids from casein are absorbed more slowly so that blood levels are elevated over a long period of time. After resistance exercise, muscles take up similar amounts of amino acids from casein and whey.

Ingesting other energy sources in combination with protein also affects how rapidly the whole body and skeletal muscles take up amino acids. At rest, the body seems to retain more amino acids when the protein is con-

sumed with CHO. Also, CHO ingestion improves the use of amino acids when they are ingested together after resistance exercise. Importantly, a small amount of the essential amino acids together is more effective than large amounts of protein. The timing of protein ingestion is critical.

Finally, it is unreasonable to give broad recommendations for a particular amount of protein for Warfighters given all the important regulating and interacting factors. However, more is **not** better.

Vitamin and Mineral Needs

Currently, the micronutrient requirements for endurance training are not well defined. Because of the nature of your training, daily overall needs may be 1.5–3 times greater than the average man. If a healthy diet composed of a variety of different foods that meets your energy requirements is consumed, daily vitamin and mineral needs should be met (see Chapter 4 for information on food sources of various vitamins and minerals). Because endurance exercise may increase the need for antioxidants due to increases in free radical exposure and cellular breakdown, it is recommended that several foods rich in natural antioxidants (vitamin C, vitamin E and beta carotene) be consumed, as shown in the table below.

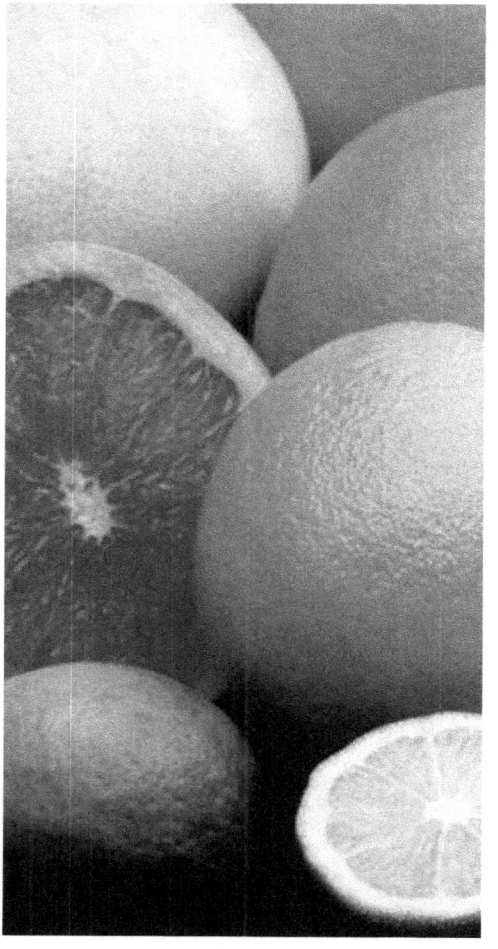

Table 9–3. Some Good Food Sources of Selected Antioxidant Nutrients		
Vitamin C	**Vitamin E**	**Carotenoids**
Orange juice	Sunflower seeds	Carrots
Grapefruit juice	Wheat germ	Spinach
Broccoli	Almonds	Cantaloupe
Orange	Peanuts	Broccoli
Strawberries	Spinach	Winter squash
Cauliflower	Olive oil	Dried apricots
Red, yellow peppers	Tomato	Sweet potatoes
Papaya	Kiwi	Mango
Dried berries	Mango	Pumpkin

One important consideration is electrolyte (sodium and potassium) balance, particularly when training in hot weather. Adequate sodium is usually not a problem, unless you are on a sodium-restricted diet. However, potassium requires careful selection of foods. See Chapter 4 for good food sources of potassium for food sources of minerals.

Fluid Requirements

Ingesting fluids at regular intervals and eating foods with high water content are important for maintaining hydration and fluid status during training. Chapter 3 provides a thorough overview of fluid requirements and different types of beverages. In general:

- Drink one to two cups (8–16 oz) of water 60 minutes before a training session.

- Drink one cup (8 oz) of a 5–8% CHO drink every 30 minutes during exercise lasting more than 60 minutes. This translates into 50–80 grams of CHO/Liter or 9–19 grams/8 oz (Read the Nutrition Label to determine the amount of CHO per serving).

- To avoid stomach cramps, beverages with a CHO content over 8%, such as undiluted fruit juices, most energy drinks, and regular sodas, should not be ingested during exercise.

- Commercial fluid replacement beverages or diluted juices are recommended during training session lasting over 60 minutes.

- Beverages consumed after prolonged exercise should contain sodium, potassium, and CHO.

It is possible to drink too much water.

Water intoxication is a concern among Warfighters and other athletes who sustain long bouts of exercise without replenishing important electrolytes contained in sports drinks, gels, and blocks. When drinking plain water (without sodium), blood levels of sodium may become low and result in "hyponatremia," or low blood sodium. This condition is associated with severe headaches, diarrhea and nausea and, potentially, convulsions and death.

Nutritional Interventions for Endurance

Nutritional manipulations/interventions can delay fatigue and prevent conditions detrimental to health and performance such as low blood sugar, dehydration, and low blood sodium. The primary interventions include:

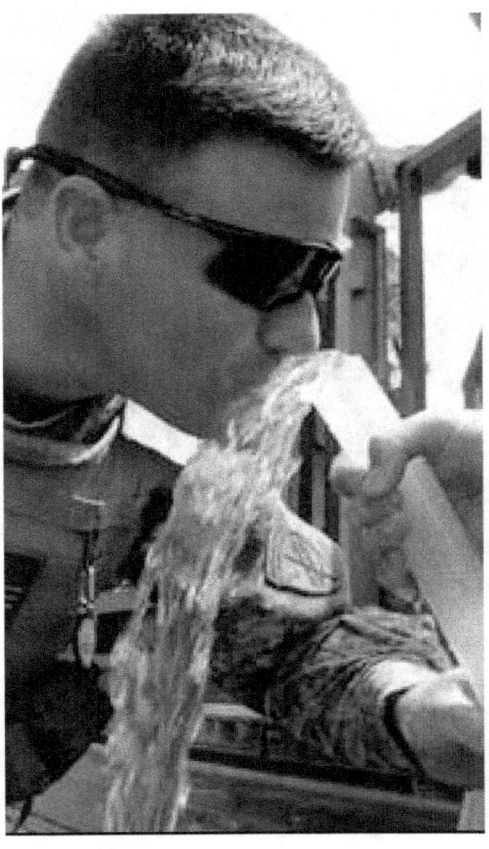

- Drinking 1–2 cups of a CHO beverage (5-8%) with electrolytes every 30 minutes during exercise to maintain performance.

- When an activity has been maintained for 2–3 hours without a CHO source, blood glucose levels will fall and cause fatigue. Ingestion of CHO beverages will prevent the fall in blood sugar (glucose) and delay fatigue. Ingesting CHO **after** exhaustion will not allow immediate resumption of activities.

- Solid CHO foods, such as fruits, and energy and sports bars, are acceptable during exercise, provided they are tolerated. Food selections are personal choices, but some foods may cause stomach cramps and diarrhea if eaten during exercise. Dietary fiber intake should be limited during endurance exercise to avoid gastrointestinal discomfort and possible pitstops in the woods for relief. All foods used for replenishment during sustained operations and exercise sessions should be "familiar" foods.

Dietary manipulations should be tested during training to ensure they are tolerated during operations.

"I've seen firsthand how the combination of core physical training and proper nutrition enable [Warfighters] to take an unbelievable beating, stay mentally sharp, and accomplish the mission over long ranges in incredible sea states; and then do it again the next night."

CAPT Kent Paro, USN
Former CO NSWSBT20

10 Bulking Up

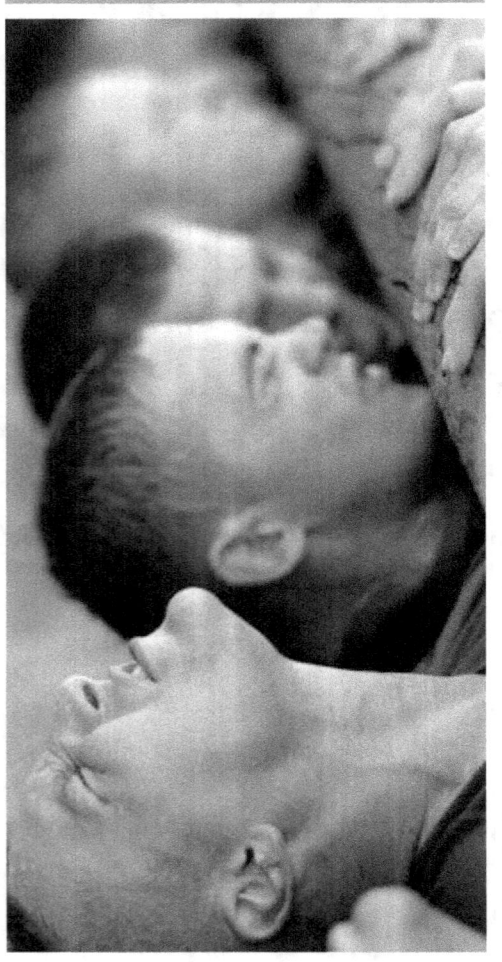

Key Points

• Proper and consistent strength training, adequate rest and a balanced diet will provide the lasting **edge** when it comes to building strength and muscle mass.

• Eating a wide variety of foods and matching energy intake with energy output will provide optimal nutrition for building muscle.

• All Warfighters require no more than 1 gram of protein per pound of body weight per day.

• Adequate amounts of fluids are vital to muscle metabolism and contractility.

• Spend money on "real" foods, **not** supplements and protein powders.

Military missions and training require strength. A strength training program enhances physical conditioning, builds functional strength and allows you to perform and complete strenuous missions. The appropriate strength training program combined with a well planned nutritional strategy can also help optimize performance and prevent musculoskeletal injuries. In this chapter, information on strength training and the unique dietary requirements for this training will be provided.

Benefits of Strength Training

Strength training should complement endurance training workouts. The specific benefits of strength training include:

• Increased muscle strength and endurance.

• Increased muscle fiber size.

• Increased ligament and tendon strength.

• Greater protection against "overuse" injury.

Because strength training makes you stronger, the risk of injuries that may accompany endurance training is reduced. Finally, strength training can make you faster at tasks requiring short bursts of activity.

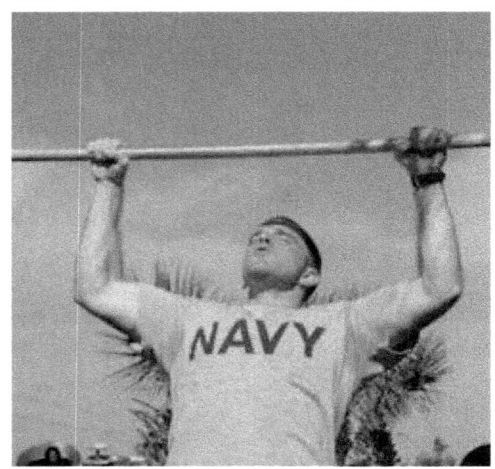

Factors Determining Muscle Mass

Skeletal muscle accounts for over 50% of body weight and is very important in terms of regulating metabolism. The mechanical and metabolic demands imposed on skeletal muscle require a constant "remodeling," or breaking down and rebuilding of various muscle proteins that support muscle contraction (structural) and muscle metabolism (functional). This remodeling is critical to maintain and ensure muscle quality—if proteins were not constantly being broken down, damaged proteins would prevail. Various factors regulate the balance between breaking down and building up, as well as the quantity and quality, of proteins. Some factors, like genetics, are out of our control, but two major "controllable" factors that participate in regulating muscle "remodeling" are:

- **Exercise:** Resistance training increases muscle mass by promoting the turnover and re-build-up of structural proteins.

- **Nutritional Status:** Nutrients for muscle growth shift the balance from "breaking down" to "building up."

Principles of Training

For functional fitness, the importance of specificity, overload and progression must be considered.

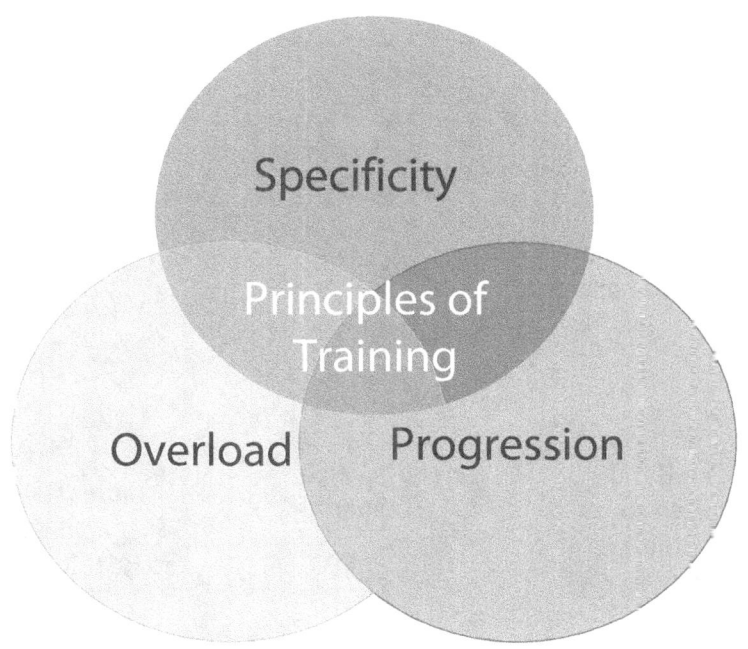

- **Specificity:** Demands placed on the body will dictate the type of adaptation that occurs.

- **Overload:** Increasing the intensity of training by increasing the number of sessions per week, performing more difficult exercises, adding weight or sets of exercise, and/or decreasing rest periods between exercise sets increases the load.

- **Progression:** Gradual increases in the load/intensity.

When these important principles are integrated into the physical training program, positive outcomes and fewer injuries can be expected. In addition, a 5–10 minute aerobic warm-up period is advised to increase blood flow to the muscles and get the motor neurons firing.

Once muscular strength is achieved, optimal muscular endurance should be pursued.

Lifting Pitfalls to Poor Performance

Although muscle strength and development are a part of a Warfighter's physical training, moderation is the key, and recommended for balancing strength and maintaining cardiovascular fitness. Heavy lifting is common for Warfighters because carrying and lifting heavy objects is important operationally; however, there are disadvantages to **only** lifting heavy weights.

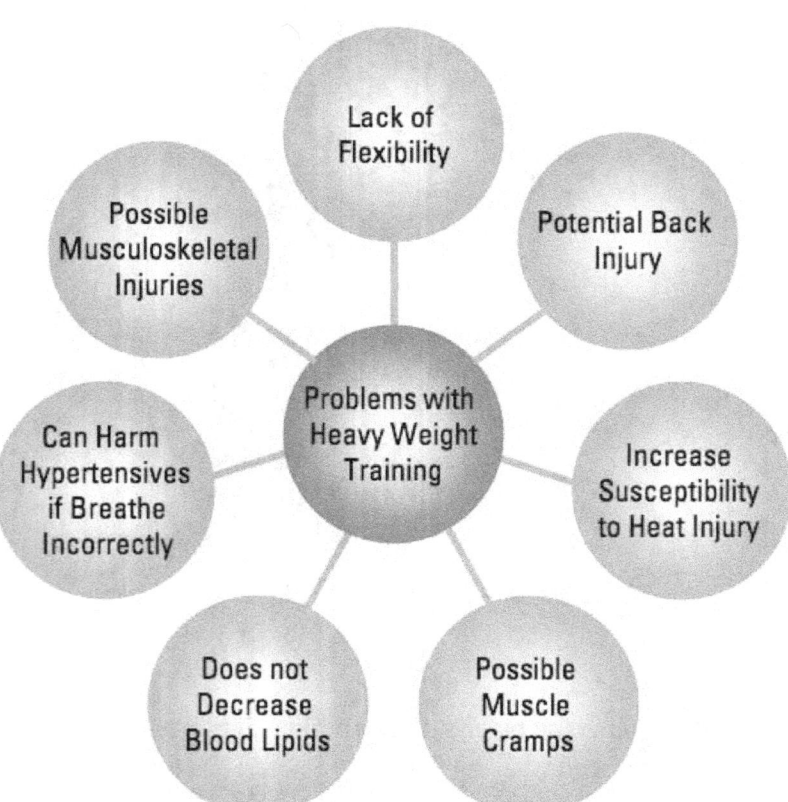

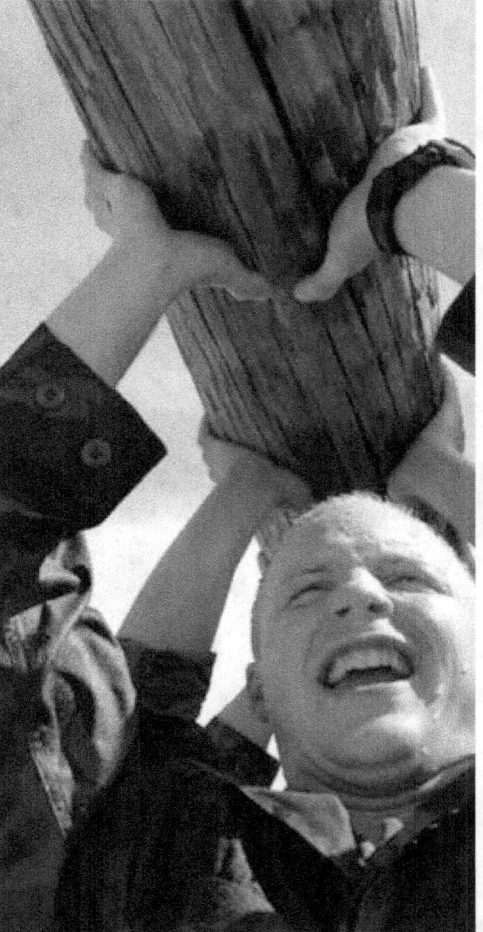

The major pitfall is that heavy weight lifting can limit range of motion and strengthens **only** the muscles within that specific range.

Resistance and endurance exercise *must* be combined for injury prevention and performance optimization.

Range of Motion

Taking a muscle through its full range of motion is critical. Full-range of motion movements contract and strengthen the primary muscles you're working and stretch the opposing (antagonist) muscles. This contributes to both muscle strength and joint flexibility.

Weight training strengthens the muscle when it goes through the full range of motion.

It is important to remember that proper form and alignment are required when using any strength training equipment to maximize safety. Certified Strength and Conditioning Specialists (CSCS) are very useful for developing the appropriate functional lifting routines and tailoring a training program consistent with individual operational tempos.

Equipment Considerations

Resistance training programs should be individualized to meet specific training goals. To achieve training goals, the different types of strength training equipment must be considered. Free weights (dumbbells, barbells and kettle bells) and ground-based equipment, which are used in many military training sites, require more coordination because of requirements for muscular balance, control, and stabilization. Free weights mimic real life movements, in that there is no "fixed" range of motion. Multiple muscles work together in order to achieve form and technique.

In contrast to free weights, various weight machines, such as Nautilus, Cybex, LifeFitness and BodyMaster, can be used without a spotter, and correct form is achieved easily, which increases the safety factor. However, many machines do not take the muscles through the full range of motion. Machines for leg curls (hamstrings) and leg extensions (quadriceps) are ones that do allow a full range of motion.

Example:

Train 3 hrs each day and take in 3,500 kcal/day

60% of energy from CHO = 3,500 x 0.60 = 2,100 kcal from CHO

Amount of CHO = 2,100/4 kcal = 525 grams of CHO

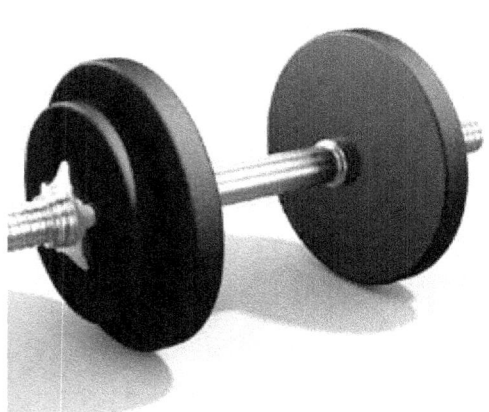

Training Features of Free Weights

Offers numerous movement planes and hand positions.

Safety and ease of use.

Use of stabilizing muscles.

Fixed range of motion.

Mimics real life movement.

Rotational resistance.

Victims of Bigorexia

Bigorexia, or muscle dysmorphia, is an obsession about being muscular; it is the opposite of anorexia. Preoccupation with becoming more muscular may lead to exercising even when in pain or with an injury, being compulsive about training every day and refusing to take a day off, skipping social events for training, and/or refusing to go to restaurants, parties, or social gatherings that offer food in order to remain on a strict nutritional regimen. The bottom line is that victims of bigorexia are never accepting of their bodies: it is never muscular enough. Excessive training is not the only repercussion. Other symptoms of bigorexia are:

- Spending excessive amounts on supplements.

- Using steroids to increase muscle mass.

- Being unhappy with one's physique.

The need for spotters when lifting very heavy free weights is important.

Protein Requirements for Strength Training

The protein needs of strength and endurance athletes are quite similar: 0.6–0.9 grams of protein per pound body weight each day will meet all Warfighters' daily protein requirements. However, many Warfighters believe that more protein is better. In fact, more may **compromise** the quality of the protein. Protein intakes above 1.6 grams per pound per day may inhibit muscle growth, increase loss of calcium, and compromise bone health. It is not the amount, but rather the quality of the protein and effectiveness of the strength training workout that determine muscle mass.

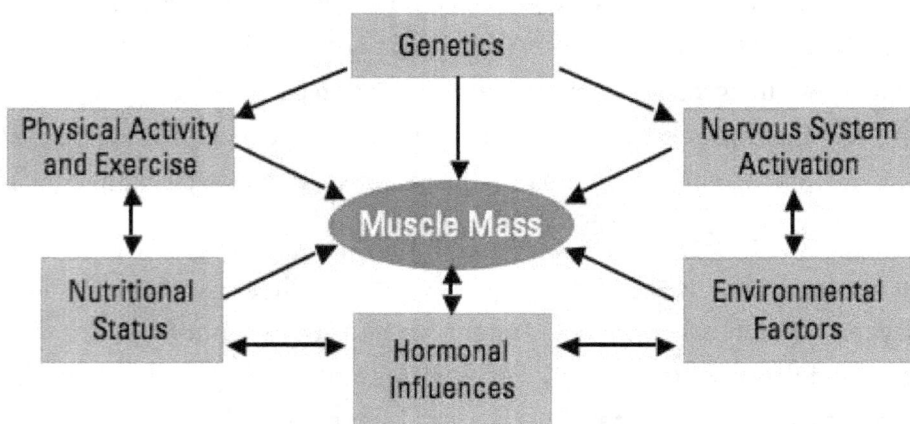

Protein intakes over 1.6 g/pound each day may compromise appropriate anabolic signals that promote muscle growth.

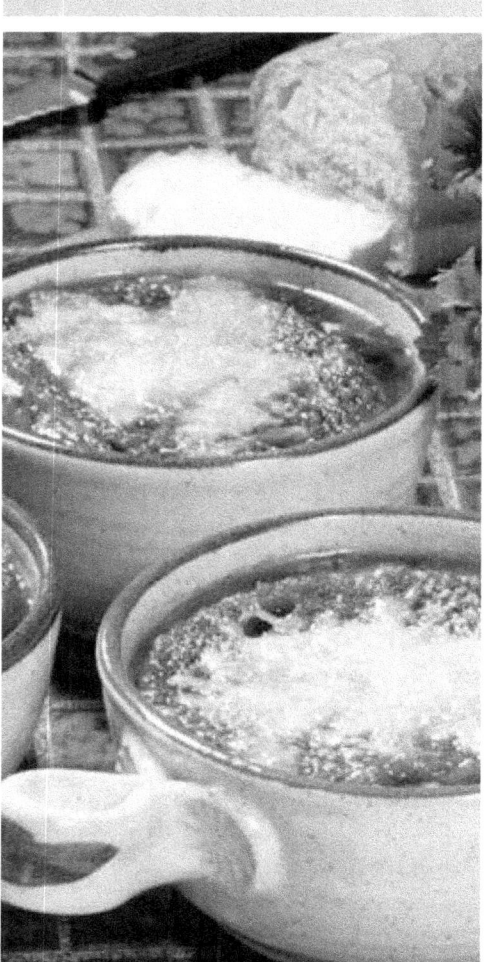

Table 10–1 provides an overview of calculating protein requirements and Table 10–2 presents the protein content of commonly eaten foods. Some foods with high quality proteins are:

- Chicken breast, 8 oz.

- Sirloin Steak, 8 oz.

- Subway Turkey Sub.

- Subway Roast Beef Sub.

Table 10–1. How to Calculate Protein Requirements

How Much Protein Do I Need?

175 lbs x 0.9 grams =	158 grams
175 lbs x 0.6 grams =	105 grams
Body Weight x Requirement	Grams/Day

My Protein Requirements Are:

_____ x 0.8 grams = _____

_____ x 0.6 grams = _____

Body Weight x Requirement	Grams/Day

Table 10–2. Examples of Where You Get Protein			
Food Item	Protein (g)	Food Item	Protein (g)
Chicken Breast (8 oz)	72	Sirloin Steak (8 oz)	62
Subway Roast Beef Sub	41	Subway Turkey Sub	42
Vanilla Milkshake	9	Chili (8 oz bowl)	19
Egg McMuffin, 1	18	Sports Bar, 1	12
TOTAL	138	TOTAL	135

Most American diets provide more protein than shown in the example, since protein is also in milk, cheese, fish, and non-animal sources of foods (whole grains, beans, and pasta). Most athletes also consume additional protein in commercially available sports bars, protein powders or carbohydrate/protein supplements.

Muscle is only 20% protein and the rest is water and minerals, lactic acid, urea and high-energy phosphates, so it is clear that eating a high protein diet in order to bulk up just doesn't add up!

Protein supplements, which provide excessive amounts of protein or selected amino acids, are discouraged. Although heavily advertised, and in some cases endorsed by celebrities, very high protein intakes from supplements are **not** needed to build muscle. A properly balanced diet can meet your protein needs very effectively.

Concerns with High Protein Intakes

The extra dietary protein must be broken down, which results in increased formation and excretion of the waste product, "urea." This additional waste increases fluid requirements, and places a considerable load on the liver and kidneys. In extreme cases, excessive protein intakes can result in kidney failure. In some individuals, high protein intakes can cause:

- Hypertension.
- Increased fluid needs.
- Diarrhea/abdominal cramps.
- Imbalance of the essential amino acids.

If 100 extra grams of protein were eaten every day for one week, muscle mass should increase by 7 pounds! *Clearly*, this is not the case.

Other Nutritional Requirements

Carbohydrate Requirements

Strength training relies on glycogen stores for energy. Thus, carbohydrates (CHO) are very important.

50–70% of daily energy intake should come from CHO.

The CHO recommendations for strength training are somewhat less than for endurance athletes, since the overall energy requirements of weight lifting are less. However, depending on the training schedule and aerobic workout duration, 2.5–4 grams of CHO per pound body weight per day may be needed. If only protein is eaten, the body must work hard

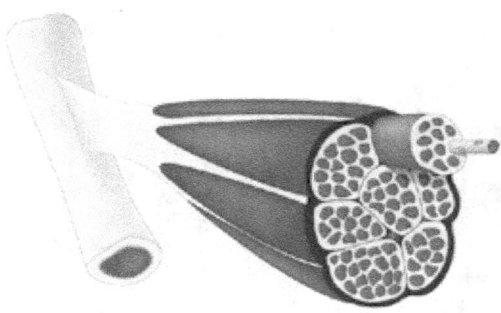

Protein 20%
Water 75%
Inorganic Salts, Urea, Lactate 5%

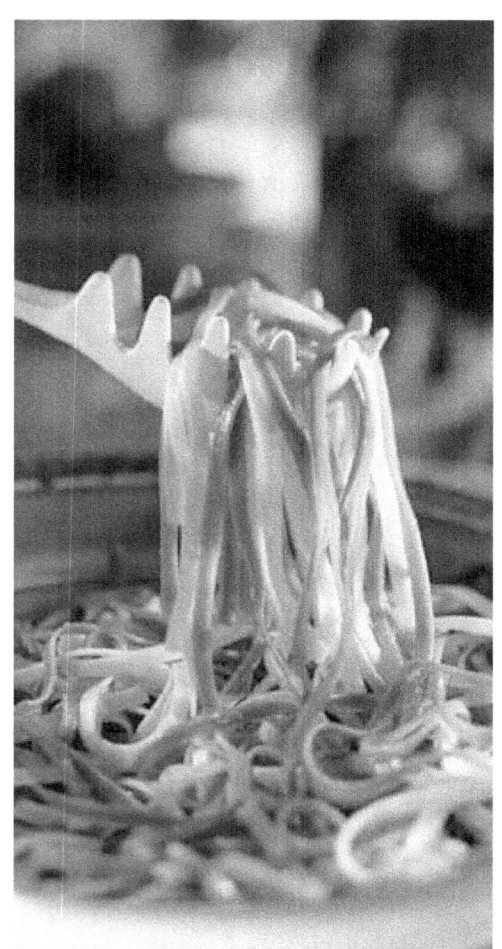

Resistance training for muscle mass gains requires more focused attention on positive energy balance than protein intake.

to convert protein into glucose, which is required by the brain and muscles for fuel.

Carbohydrate is the primary fuel source for strength training.

Fat Requirements

A thorough discussion of fat was provided in Chapter 3, but for fats in general, the recommendation is:

Less than 35% of your energy should come from fat.

Remember, less than 10% of the fat should come from saturated fat and the balance from mono- and poly-unsaturated fats.

Vitamins and Minerals

If you meet your daily energy needs from a variety of different foods, you should be able to meet your vitamin and mineral needs. See Chapter 4 for information on food sources of various vitamins and minerals.

Dietary Considerations for Bulking-Up

The major stimulus for muscle growth and strength are weight training and appropriately timed, good nutrition. After weight training, nutrient dense energy sources are the single most important factor that affects muscle gain—you must have the energy to train effectively on a daily basis. All too often, Warfighters are exhausted by the long Friday workouts, due to not eating regularly and consistently over the week. Such dietary habits are not conducive to building muscle mass.

If nutrient intake is lacking as a result of poor meal planning and/or high operational tempo, skeletal muscle may be in a negative protein balance or a catabolic state. For optimal muscle remodeling and growth, the timing and type of nutrients are critical. Appropriate nutritional interventions immediately after the exercise and over the next 24 hours are essential for maintaining and promoting muscle mass.

Table 10–3. Nutritional Tips for Bulking-Up

Break for breakfast. Consume a hearty breakfast containing whole grains, fruit, and protein from lean meats and eggs, as well as low-fat dairy products.

Graze frequently throughout the day. Keep a supply of healthy snacks to help replenish muscle glycogen.

Don't go without food for more than 4 hours (if possible) to avoid glycogen depletion.

Remember "CPF" meal planning: Eat at least 3 of the 5 food groups—a mixed meal containing CHO, protein and fat—for an optimal fueling strategy to maintain energy for strong and effective strength trainings. Some combinations are:	Fish, rice, and vegetables
	Cereal, milk, and fruit
	Turkey on whole grain bread with tomato, lettuce, and onion
	Low-fat yogurt, grape nuts and fruit
	Vegetable burrito (tortilla, vegetables and cheese)
Avoid amino acid supplementation and minimize protein powders—real foods are more nutrient-dense. Good food sources of proteins include:	Lean beef, lamb, and pork
	Low-fat dairy
	Fish
	Poultry
	Venison

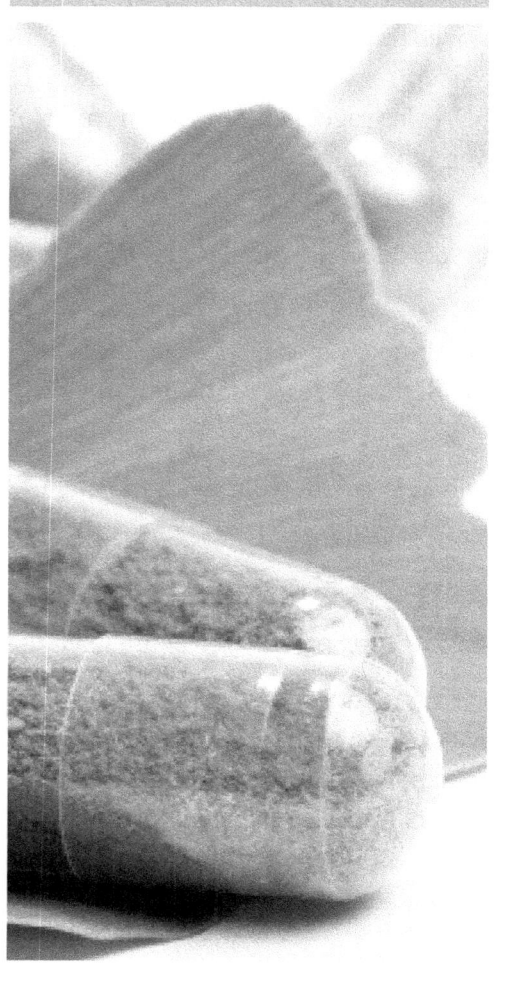

11 Looking for the Edge— Dietary Supplements

Key Points

- Dietary supplements (DS) sold on military installations are not always safe, effective or legal.

- Manufacturers of DS are not required to conduct research on safety or effectiveness. The Food and Drug Administration must prove a product is unsafe before it can be taken off the market.

- If you use DS, select high quality products with USP (United States Pharmacopeia) certification labels. The label assures consumers that the product has been tested and verified in terms of its ingredients and manufacturing process.

- Combining and stacking of DS increases the potential for undesired and unsafe side effects.

- Energy drinks are not regulated and the long-term effects of their combined ingredients are unknown.

The most common reasons active duty personnel give for using DS include improving performance, increasing muscle mass, enhancing energy level, accelerating recovery, increasing alertness, boosting their immune system, and improving joint function. The best sources of information on DS are dietitians, sports nutritionists, physicians, or pharmacists. The purpose of this chapter is to provide an overview of dietary supplements, describe issues with dietary supplements, and provide basic information on a number of commonly used supplements. This will not be inclusive as new products appear on a regular basis, but the information is for educational purposes.

Individuals who spend their money on supplements should be aware that these products target our human desire for health and performance shortcuts. Some may be detrimental and dangerous: if it sounds too good to be true, it probably is. The consequences of taking various supplements, either alone or in combination, should be carefully considered, and the information obtained for making that decision should be from reputable sources.

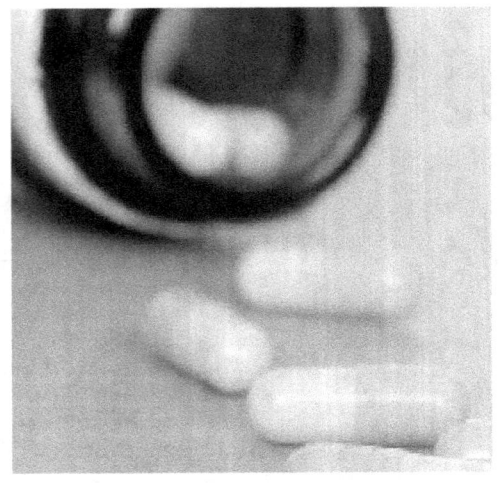

Purity is a concern: Supplements may be contaminated with heavy metals and even prescription medications.

Dietary Supplements and the Law

Well over 50% of the US population take some type of dietary supplements. Sales of vitamins, minerals, herbs, meal supplements, sports-nutrition supplements, and specialty supplements were in excess of $22 billion in 2006. To understand why dietary supplement use is a concern, one must appreciate the history. In 1994 the Dietary Supplement Health and Education Act (DSHEA) was passed by Congress for several reasons:

- Limit impediments to marketing and promoting dietary supplements.

- Provide for wide availability of supplements to consumers.

- Enhance information available to consumers.

The passing of DSHEA gave the Food and Drug Administration (FDA) regulatory control over dietary supplements, and the law required that the label of a dietary supplement provide the name and quantity of each ingredient. However, it is incumbent upon the manufacturer to provide the information and the innocent consumer assumes that information on labels is truthful and not misleading. This is, more than often, not the case. ConsumerLab.com, a product-certification company, conducted a survey of nearly 1,000 supplements and found that one in four had quality problems.

The FDA also regulates whether new ingredients can enter the marketplace or existing ones should be removed for safety reasons. However, federal rules requiring makers of dietary supplements to test all their ingredients were not part of DSHEA. The FDA also regulates what claims may (or may not) be made, but they do not monitor claims. The regulations within DSHEA contain many gaps. Some of the concerns include:

- The responsibility of ensuring that products are properly labeled lies with the manufacturer.

- Supplement ingredients sold in the United States before October 15, 1994 are presumed to be safe and are therefore not subject to review by the FDA for safety.

- The responsibility of providing evidence of safety lies with the manufacturer.

- The FDA has to prove that a product is not safe if it is already on the market.

- Government resources to check dietary supplement quality are limited.

In June, 2007, FDA imposed new regulations, which had been mandated by DSHEA. The FDA established regulations that dietary supplements must be produced in a quality manner, do not contain contaminants or impurities, and are accurately labeled. Supplement manufacturers will now be required to test all of the ingredients in their products to make sure they are neither adulterated nor contaminated.

Combining and Stacking Supplements

Once it is known what a supplement contains, consideration should be given to what might happen when multiple supplements are combined, or "stacked." The concept of "stacking" is a concern. Many variations of "stacking" exist. Several examples of stacking and how they work are listed:

- "Additive," or, 1+1=2. This suggests that when two supplements are combined, the effect is equal to the sum of the individual effects. An example of this concept might include calcium and vitamin D.

- "Antagonize," or, 1+1=0. In this case, the effects of one supplement may actually negate the effects of another. One example is the combination of creatine and caffeine: Studies have shown that caffeine antagonizes the effects of creatine.

- "Synergize," or, 1+1=3. This is seen when two supplements are combined and their effect is greater than the sum of their individual effects. An example is Coenzyme Q10 and fat: When CoQ10 is taken with fat, the action of CoQ10 exceeds what is would be if not taken with fat.

- "Potentiate," or, 1+1=10 is similar to synergism, but to a much greater degree. Two examples are vitamin C and iron, and ginseng and caffeine. Vitamin C enhances the absorption of iron, which is a good thing, but if ginseng is taken with caffeine, it may be detrimental, as ginseng has been shown to increase the effects of caffeine, to possibly cause nervousness, sweating, insomnia, and/or an irregular heartbeat.

The number of potential stacking combinations is staggering and the effects of combinations of ingredients are, for the most part, unknown. One stacking approach that has proven deadly is the "EAC" stack, with ephedra, aspirin and caffeine. Now that ephedra is banned, ephedra-free products are being used, but the combination remains dangerous and should be avoided.

A list of products commonly considered "stackers" is shown on the following page. Some are trade names and many are potentially dangerous. Become familiar with ingredients and ask questions about combining different compounds.

Table 11–1. Common "Stackers"	
Muscle Milk	A blend of casein and whey proteins, combined with fats and other substances.
NO2 or NO	Products contain many ingredients, but typically arginine (described below).

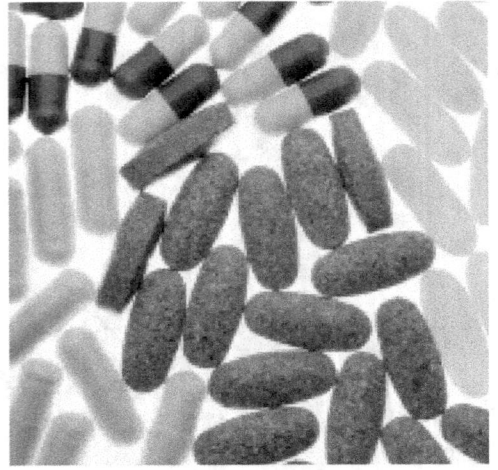

Table 11–1. Common "Stackers"	
Hydroxycut	A classic EAC stacker that has resulted in a number of deaths: **Avoid.**
GAKIC	A NO product with Glycine-l-arginine-alpha-ketoisocaproic acid.
Epovar	A NO product with Magnesium Orotate and Potassium Orotate.
Zantrex 3	A thermogenic product with many forms of caffeine.
Xenadrine EFX	A thermogenic product with synephrine and many forms of caffeine. Company was fined for false advertising.
Triflex	A combination of glucosamine, chondroitin and methylsulfonyl-methane.
Arginine Ethyl Ester	A NO product.
Redline	A line of products high in caffeine and other substances.
ZMA	A combination of vitamin B6. Magnesium and Zinc, among other ingredients.
Lipo-Products (Lipo-6, Lipo-AMP, Lipo-THIN Lipo-Complex)	Contains many combinations of ingredients—thermogenic agent.
Animal Cuts	May contain up to 20 ingredients, including synephrine: **Avoid.**
Metabolic XXX (Drive, Booster, Action, or Optimizer)	Contains many combinations of ingredients—thermogenic agent: **Avoid.**

Be a Smart Shopper: Consumer Safety Tips

Supplements should be clearly labeled with "Seals of Approval." The seals include "CL" for a Consumer Lab seal of approval and "USP" for US Pharmacopoeia. These for-profit and not-for-profit agencies inspect the product and assign scores or ratings if they contain no contaminants, have standardized doses, can be absorbed by the body, can be broken down by the body, and the company that produces the products has quality control standards in place during production and manufacturing to ensure safety and purity.

If supplements do not have approval
seals, do not use them!

Individual Products Discussed

It would be impossible to discuss all of the dietary supplements and herbals available. However, some are used more than others. Although not inclusive, the following products will be discussed:

Bitter Orange	Boron	Branched Chain Amino Acids
Caffeine	Carnitine	Choline
Chondroitin Sulfate	Chromium	Chrysin
CoEnzyme Q10	Conjugated Linoleic Acid	Cordyceps
Creatine	DHEA	Ephedra
Fish Oil	Ginkgo Biloba	Ginseng
Glucosamine	Glutamine	Guarana
HMB	Hoodia	Hydroxycitric Acid/ HCA

Hydroxymethylbu-tyrate	5-Hydroxytrypto-phan	Lysine
Melatonin	Nitric Oxide	Pycnogenol
Quercetin	St. John's Wort	Synephrine
Tribulus Terrestris	Tryptophan	Turmeric
Tyrosine	Whey Protein	Yohimbe

Products that are lightly shaded should not be used.

Performance-Enhancing Agents

Performance enhancing agents are substances claiming to increase work output, performance or lean muscle mass. A discussion of each is not possible, so some that are mass marketed are discussed.

Muscle Building Agents

These agents are listed in alphabetical order.

Boron

Claims	Builds muscles and increases testosterone levels; may enhance cognitive function.
Other Names	Borate, Boric Acid, Boric Tartrate, and Sodium Borate.
How It Works	No one is sure how (or if) boron is effective because its biological role is unknown.
Dose	No DRI has been established for boron, but a diet high in boron would provide approximately 3.25 mg boron per 2,000 kcal/day, whereas a diet low in boron would provide less than 0.25 mg boron per 2,000 kcal/day. The maximum dose, at which no adverse effects would be expected, is 20 mg per day for adults.
Adverse Effects	None have been reported.

Boron

Comments   More evidence is needed to determine the importance of boron.

L-Carnitine

Claims   Enhance athletic performance, particularly endurance.

Other Names   Carnitine, Carnitor, DL-Carnitine, L-Carnitine Fumarate, L-Carnitine L-Tartrate, L-Carnitine Tartrate, Levocarnitine, Levocarnitine Fumurate.

How It Works   Carnitine enhances the transport of fats to the energy powerhouse within the muscle and the subsequent use of fats as fuel during exercise.

Dose   2–4 grams/day have been taken without any clear benefit. No dose has been established for improving athletic performance.

Adverse Effects   Nausea, vomiting, cramps, diarrhea, heartburn, body odor, and seizures have been reported, when used inappropriately.

Comments   Carnitine is found naturally in the body and can be obtained in the diet from red meats and dairy products. Taking L-Carnitine has **not** been shown to improve athletic performance or endurance.

Chromium

Claims   Increases lean muscle mass; is the natural alternative to steroids.

Other Names   Chromium Acetate, Chromium Chloride, Chromium Nicotinate, Chromium Picolinate, Chromium Polynicotinate, Chromium Proteinate, Chromium Trichloride, Chromium Tripicolinate, Cr3+, Glucose Tolerance Factor-Cr, GTF, GTF Chromium, GTF-Cr.

Chromium

How It Works	Chromium is part of a number of substances that regulate glucose metabolism.
Dose	Doses ranging from 200–1000 mcg/day appear to be safe.
Adverse Effects	Chromium can cause headache, insomnia, and motor dysfunction in some people in doses as low as 200–400 mcg/day.
Comments	Some evidence suggests that chromium can increase weight loss, body fat loss and increase lean body mass in people taking chromium picolinate (200–400 mcg/day) as part of a resistance training program, but the results are questionable. Chromium may be helpful in diabetes, hypertension, and potentially weight loss.

Chrysin

Claims	Enhances response to resistance training.
Other Names	Flavone X, Flavonoid, Galangin Flavanone.
How It Works	Claims are that it increases testosterone levels.
Dose	A dose of 300 mg daily has been used, but it is usually in combination with other potential testosterone releasers, such as DHEA, Tribulus terrestris, and saw palmetto.
Adverse Effects	None have been reported.
Comments	Chrysin is a naturally occurring isoflavone found in various plants. Most chrysin products are extracted from the passion flower species. It does not seem to be effective for enhancing the response to resistance training in athletes, but minimal data are available for this herbal because it is typically used in combination with other substances.

Creatine

Claims

Gain muscle mass and improve anaerobic performance.

Other Names

Creatine Monohydrate, Creatine Citrate, Creatine Ethyl Ester, Creatine Ethyl Ester HCl, Serum Creatine, Creatine Pyruvate, Phosphocreatine.

How It Works

Taking creatine allows the muscles to store greater amounts of creatine phosphate (or phosphocreatine), which is used to regenerate ATP, the primary energy for muscle contraction. Creatine can cause visible bulking up of muscles by increasing the water content of muscle cells.

Dose

A dose of 3 grams/day is adequate and a loading dose is unnecessary. The dose commonly recommended for loading is 20 grams/day for 5 days followed by a maintenance dose of less than 10 grams/day. The higher doses are not any more effective than the 3 grams/day.

Adverse Effects

Side effects, not demonstrated by research but reported in association with creatine use include: muscle cramping, gastrointestinal disturbances, kidney problems or dehydration. High doses of creatine may negatively affect kidney function. Individuals taking drugs that affect the kidneys (cyclosporine, gentamicin, tobramycin, and NSAIDS; ibuprofen and naproxen) should avoid high doses of creatine. Caffeine may negate the effects of creatine.

Comments

The body makes creatine (1–2 gm/day) with 95% being stored in skeletal muscle. Creatine supplementation may produce a small increase in explosive strength or enhance performance for short burst, high-intensity activities, like weight lifting and sprinting. It does not improve endurance and if weight gain is high, endurance may be impaired.

HMB (Hydroxymethylbutyrate)

Claims Increases muscle mass and enhances recovery.

Other Names B-Hydroxy B-Methylbutyrate Monohydrate, Beta-Hydroxy-Beta-Methylbutyric Acid, Hydroxymethyl Butyrate.

How It Works HMB might promote muscle growth by decreasing or slowing down the catabolism or breakdown of muscle protein.

Dose Doses of 1 gram three times daily or 1.5 grams once or twice daily have been used for muscle building and increasing strength during weight training.

Adverse Effects No known adverse effects have been linked to HMB.

Comments Evidence about the effectiveness of HMB for weight training is conflicting. Some research shows no effect and other data suggest that HMB may be effective in people who have not previously trained. HMB is a by-product of the metabolism of the amino acid, leucine and a precursor to cholesterol.

Nitric Oxide (NO)

Claims Enhances delivery of nutrients to muscles so they can increase in mass with training. Increases strength, improves in stamina, and accelerates recovery.

Other Names NO-Xplode, Nitrix, NOX-CG3, NOx2, and NO.

How It Works NO works in part by increasing bloods flow. However, supplements marketed as NO do not contain NO because it is a gas, which cannot be put into a pill. Rather the products contain the amino acid, arginine.

Nitric Oxide (NO)

Dose
No dose has been established. Products marketed as NO will vary with the type and amount of ingredients.

Adverse Effects
Because NO products are all different, it is very difficult to document adverse effects. Combinations of ingredients are a concern.

Comments
Nitric Oxide is actually a gas produced in the body from the amino acid, arginine, to communicate with other cells. Most NO products are typically amino acid mixtures containing arginine alpha-ketoglutarate (A-AKG) and arginine-ketoisocaproate (A-KIC).

Tribulus Terrestris

Claims
Enhances muscle strength and athletic performance; an antidote for male impotence.

Other Names
Cat's-Head, Devil's-Thorn, Devil's-Weed, Goathead, Nature's Viagra, Puncture Weed, Tribule Terrestre.

How It Works
Increases levels of testosterone, dehydroepiandrosterone (DHEA), and dihydrotestosterone.

Dose
A dose of 250 mg per day has been used.

Adverse Effects
None have been reported.

Comments
No study to date has demonstrated any benefit to strength or athletic performance after taking Tribulus Terrestris. This herbal is derived from a Mediterranean plant that bears a spine-covered fruit.

Athletic/Recovery Agents

The list of substances marketed to enhance or improve athletic performance is extensive and continually changing. Some commonly used products, listed in alphabetical order (not order of effectiveness), are described below.

Branched-Chain Amino Acids (BCAA)

Claims	Enhances exercise performance, prevents fatigue, reduces protein and muscle breakdown during intense exercise.
Other Names	BCAA, Isoleucine, Leucine, L-Isoleucine, L-Leucine, L-Valine, N-Acetyl Leucine, Valine.
How It Works	BCAA act as signaling molecules to stimulate protein synthesis or production; they are also used as an energy source during stress.
Dose	No established dose.
Adverse Effects	BCAA in doses of 60 grams or higher daily can increase ammonia levels in the blood, which can lead to fatigue and loss of motor coordination.
Comments	Research has not demonstrated that BCAA enhance exercise or athletic performance. The Estimated Average Requirements for BCAA are 68–144 mg/kg/day (leucine 34 mg/day; isoleucine 15 mg/day; valine 19 mg/day). This would equate to 4.7–10 grams per day for a 70 kg (154 lb) person. BCAA are found in meat, dairy foods, and legumes. About 15–25% of the total dietary protein intake is BCAA.

Caffeine

Claims	Improves mental alertness and enhances athletic performance; used for weight loss and diabetes.
Other Names	Methylxanthines and herbal products such as Black Tea, Green Tea, Oolong Tea, Coffee, Cola Nut, Guarana, and Maté.

Caffeine

How It Works

Caffeine is a stimulant. It stimulates the central nervous system, heart, skeletal muscles, and respiration.

Dose

100-600 mg/day consumed over a period of 4–8 hours is the most common dose. For endurance doses may range from 2-10 mg per kg body weight. Higher doses may produce urine levels greater than allowed by the International Olympic Committee.

Adverse Effects

Adverse effects are in part determined by sensitivity to caffeine. Some people are rapid and others slow caffeine metabolizers. Reported effects of caffeine include headache, anxiety, agitation, insomnia, nervousness, restlessness, gastrointestinal distress, nausea, rapid heart rate, arrhythmias, quickened respiration, tremors, convulsions, and frequent urination. Chronic use, especially in large amounts, can produce tolerance, habituation, and psychological dependence.

Caffeine produces physical dependence and withdrawal of caffeine elicits physical and behavioral symptoms, to include:

- Headache.
- Fatigue.
- Difficulty concentrating.
- Mood disturbances (depressed mood, irritability).
- Flu-like symptoms (muscle aches, nausea, vomiting).

The symptoms of withdrawal can occur taking only 100 mg of caffeine per day for 7 days or 300 mg per day for 3 days. The onset of withdrawal symptoms occurs within 12 to 48 hours after last dose and may last up to nine days. Withdrawal symptoms, which can vary from mild to incapacitating, can be reversed 30 to 60 minutes after ingesting a product containing as little as 30 mg of caffeine.

Caffeine

Comments

Caffeine is included on the FDA list as a substance "generally recognized as safe." However, the FDA for cola beverages has established a maximum concentration for caffeine: 32.4 mg per 6 oz or 65 mg per 12 oz. Other than colas, the caffeine content of food and beverages is not regulated.

It is clear that caffeine is "performance enhancing," and because of this, the International Olympic Committee (IOC) has banned its use above a certain level (as detected in the athlete's urine). Caffeine seems to increase physical endurance and may increase the time to exhaustion. It does not seem to affect activities that require high exertion over a short period of time, such as sprinting or lifting, activity.

Comments

Caffeine improves mental performance and alertness after prolonged sleep deprivation. Some data suggest that caffeine reduces pain. Although caffeine is a diuretic, doses over 300 mg are usually required to compromise fluid status.

Some people are very sensitive to caffeine, and show symptoms (tremors, sleep disturbances, gastrointestinal upsets) after small doses. Persons who experience adverse reactions to caffeine-containing drinks or people with heart disease should avoid caffeine containing energy drinks (discussed below).

Choline

Claims

Enhance athletic performance by increasing energy and delaying fatigue in endurance activities and maintaining muscle strength for resistance exercise.

Other Names

Choline Bitartrate, Choline Chloride, Choline Citrate, Lipotropic Factor, Phosphatidylethanolamine, Alpha-GPC, Lecithin, and Phosphatidylcholine.

Choline

How It Works	Choline is an essential part of the neurotransmitter responsible for muscle contraction—acetylcholine. Maintaining a supply of choline could possibly prevent depletion of acetylcholine and sustain muscle contraction.
Dose	The typical dose is 1–2 grams/day; unsafe in amounts above 3.5 gm./day for adults over 18 years of age.
Adverse Effects	Choline can cause sweating, fishy body odor, vomiting and diarrhea.
Comments	Taking choline does not seem to enhance athletic performance or endurance or delay fatigue. However, the newer forms of choline have not been tested. Choline is a component of phosphatidylcholine or lecithin. Choline is considered a B vitamin, even though the body can make it. Liver, meat, fish, nuts, beans, eggs, and peas are high in choline. The typical diet provides 200–600 mg/day. Choline is a component of Alpha-glycerophosphorylcholine (GPC), Lecithin, and phosphatidylcholine.

Co-Enzyme Q10

Claims	Improves aerobic capacity.
Other Names	CoQ10, Coenzyme Q10, CoQ10.
How It Works	CoQ10 is important in the production of ATP and acts as an antioxidant.
Dose	A common dose is 100 mg/day divided and taken at two different times during the day. Some research suggests it might slightly improve tolerance to higher workloads, but more research is needed. No established dose has been set for aerobic performance.

Co-Enzyme Q10

Adverse Effects	None identified.
Comments	Dietary sources are meat and seafood; it can also be produced from fermenting beets and sugar cane with special strains of yeast. CoQ10 is also used for preventing "statin"-induced myopathy.

Cordyceps

Claims	Improves athletic performance, increases energy and stamina and reduces fatigue; strengthens the immune system.
Other Names	Caterpillar Fungus, Caterpillar Mushroom, Vegetable Caterpillar.
How It Works	May work by stimulating various immune cells to accelerate recovery.
Dose	Typical dose is 3 gm/day.
Adverse Effects	None identified at this time.
Comments	Cordyceps sinesis is a fungus parasite that lives on insects and arthropods. No research has demonstrated an effect on athletic performance. Many commercial products grow the parasite in the laboratory.

Ginseng

Ginseng refers to a group of extracts derived from the plant family, Araliacae. Three major types—Panax, American, and Siberian—are marketed; each are available in a variety of forms, ranging from root powders to root extracts to leaf powders and extracts. The forms also differ in terms of the active ingredients.

Claims	All forms claim to enhance resistance to environmental stress or serve as an "adaptogen", a term used to indicate that a substance strengthens the body and increases resistance to stress.

Ginseng

Claims	The name panax, or "all-healing," ginseng has been touted for a broad range of ailments and is used to restore life energy.
Other Names	• Panax ginseng (or P. ginseng) • Asian or Asiatic, Chinese, Korean, and Oriental ginseng, radix ginseng rubra, ren shen, sang, seng, red or white ginseng. Red ginseng is steamed and dried in heat or sunlight while white ginseng is simply the dried or powdered root.
Other Names	• American Ginseng (Panax quinquefolius). • Anchi Ginseng, Canadian Ginseng, Ginseng, Ginseng Root, North American Ginseng, Occidental Ginseng, Ontario Ginseng, Panax quinquefolium, Red Berry, Wisconsin Ginseng. • Siberian Ginseng (Eleutherococcus senticosus). • Acanthopanax Obovatus, Ciwujia, Ciwujia Root, Ciwujia Root Extract, Devil's Bush, Devil's Shrub, Eleuthero Ginseng, Eleuthero Root, Russian Root, Shigoka, Siberian Eleuthero, Siberian Ginseng, Thorny Bearer of Free Berries.
How It Works	Appears to work by modulating the immune system. Ginseng preparations have antioxidant properties and may lower blood glucose. Panax ginseng may work against stress by affecting the responsiveness and regulation of the stress-responsive hormone axis.
Dose	Dosing is generally around 0.6–3 grams of root powder 1 to 3 times per day for Panax ginseng as a capsule or an extract standardized to 4–8% ginsenosides, 200–600 mg/day. Dosing is slightly lower for American and Siberian ginsengs. Sometimes ginseng is taken continuously, but cycling is usually recommended. Ginseng is taken for 3 weeks to 3 months followed by 2 weeks to 2 months off.

Ginseng

Adverse Effects	Each form acts differently, but gastrointestinal, nervous, hypoglycemia, cardiovascular system effects, insomnia, slight drowsiness, anxiety, irritability, and feeling of sadness may be reported.
Comments	The form of ginseng is very important. Please read product labels—thousands of commercial products contain the various forms of Ginseng but only three are USP certified. Siberian ginseng is often misidentified or adulterated. American and Panax ginseng may be much more expensive. Be very careful when using ginseng products.
Comments	American Ginseng is indigenous to both the Americas and the Far East; it has been used as a medicinal plant for 5,000 years. Wild American ginseng is highly sought after, for that reason, it may become an endangered species in some states.

Glutamine

Claims	Enhances exercise performance and accelerates recovery from strenuous exercise.
Other Names	GLN, Glutamate, Glutamic Acid, Glutamic Acid HCl, L-Glutamic Acid, L-Glutamic Acid HCl, L-Glutamic Acid Hydrochloride, L-Glutamine, N-Acetyl-L-Glutamine.
How It Works	Glutamine works by maintaining normal function of the intestine, immune system, and muscle amino acid homeostasis during stress; it also serves as a metabolic fuel for immune cells.
Dose	Doses of 15–30 grams have been used after exercise. It appears safe at up to 40 grams/day.
Adverse Effects	None identified at this time.

Glutamine

Comments   Glutamine does not appear to enhance exercise performance; but it has been shown to suppress the rise in muscle breakdown during recovery. Importantly, glutamine may prove to be a biologic marker of overtraining.

Guarana

Claims   Enhance endurance performance, and improve mental acuity, weight loss, and reduce mental and physical fatigue.

Other Names   Brazilian Cocoa, Zoom.

How It Works   Guarana is a stimulant and contains caffeine, as well as other potentially psychoactive substances.

Dose   Doses vary, but 75 mg has been suggested. It is usually combined with other active ingredients.

Adverse Effects   Same as for caffeine.

Comments   Guarana is a plant species native to the central Amazonian Basin, with a long history of use for its stimulant effects. It is a common ingredient in Brazilian soft drinks. The guarana seed contains 3.6%–5.8% caffeine. Guarana is often used in combination with other ingredients for weight loss products and as a stimulant.

L-Lysine

Claims   Promote gains in muscle strength and mass.

Other Names   Lysine, L-Lysine HCl, Lysine Hydrochloride, Lysine Monohydrochloride.

How It Works   Lysine may stimulate the release of growth hormone.

L-Lysine

Dose	No established dose for athletic performance, but doses of 1–6 grams/day have been used, without benefit.
Adverse Effects	Can cause diarrhea and abdominal pain.
Comments	Oral doses that might be high enough to induce growth hormone (GH) release are likely to cause stomach discomfort and diarrhea. Exercise of moderate to high intensity is a far greater stimulus for GH release than lysine. No proven benefits have been established for performance, but lysine appears to be effective for reducing recurrence of herpes simplex infections.

Pycnogenol

Claims	Improves athletic endurance and decreases muscle cramps and pain.
Other Names	French Marine Pine Bark Extract, Maritime Bark Extract, OPCs, Pine Bark Extract, Pygenol.
How It Works	Benefits may reflect antioxidant activity.
Dose	Typical dose is 200 mg daily.
Adverse Effects	None identified at this time.
Comments	Pycnogenol is an extract from the bark of the French pine tree. Research has shown that it improved endurance in recreational athletes aged 20–35 yrs and prevented muscle cramps and muscular pain at rest, and pain after/during exercise.

Pyruvate

Claims	Improves athletic performance and promotes weight loss.
Other Names	Alpha-Keto Acid, Alpha-Ketopropionic Acid, Calcium Pyruvate, Calcium Pyruvate Monohydrate, Creatine Pyruvate, Magnesium Pyruvate, Potassium Pyruvate, Proacemic Acid, Pyruvic Acid, Sodium Pyruvate.
How It Works	Pyruvate serves as a metabolic regulator and may modify fat and CHO metabolism.
Dose	Doses range from 6–44 grams/day. The most effective dose has not been determined.
Adverse Effects	May cause gastric distress.
Comments	Research suggests that pyruvate, either alone or in combination with creatine, does not improve athletic performance. Its effect on weight loss remains to be determined.

Taurine

Claims	Improves mental performance and serves as an antioxidant.
Other Names	L-taurine.
How It Works	Believed to act as an antioxidant and free radical scavenger. Its presence in brain suggests it may also alter normal hormone function and neurotransmission.
Dose	A dose of 2–6 grams per day has been used.
Adverse Effects	None reported.

Taurine

Comments Taurine is a naturally occurring amino acid found in meat, fish and shellfish and is formed in the body. Dietary intakes of taurine range from 50–400 mg/day. However, taurine is now often added to energy drinks and these drinks may contain 25, 300, 2,000 mg, or 4,000 mg/L. As such, dietary intakes of taurine may be very high in individuals consuming energy drinks with added taurine. An upper limit of safety has not been determined. Taurine has not been shown to enhance performance.

Tyrosine

Claims Improves alertness following sleep deprivation; maintains cognitive performance during stress.

Other Names Acetyl-L-Tyrosine, L-tyrosine, N-Acetyl L-Tyrosine, Tyr.

How It Works Providing additional tyrosine should maintain brain tyrosine and allow continued synthesis of essential neurotransmitters and avoid negative effects of stress.

Dose Up to 150 mg/kg/day has been used to maintain alertness and cognitive performance.

Adverse Effects May cause headache, fatigue, nausea, and heartburn.

Comments Tyrosine is an amino acid made by the body from other amino acids. It is found in dairy products, meat, fish, eggs, nuts, beans, oats, and wheat. Tyrosine may improve alertness following sleep deprivation.

Whey Protein

Claims	Increase muscle mass and promote weight gain.
Other Names	Bovine Whey Protein Concentrate, Goat Milk Whey, Goat Whey, Milk Protein Isolate, Mineral Whey Concentrate, Whey, Whey Peptides, Whey Protein Concentrate, Whey Protein Hydrolysate, Whey Protein Isolate.
How It Works	May enhance immune system and regulate muscle protein synthesis.
Dose	No established dose, but from 8–30 grams per day are used. A high dose would be over 50 grams per day.
Adverse Effects	May cause nausea, thirst, bloating, cramps, fatigue, poor appetite and headache.
Comments	Whey protein is the name for a variety of proteins isolated from whey, which is the watery part of milk after milk separates into a liquid and solid phase from heating. Casein, or curds, is the protein in the solid phase. Whey protein contains carbohydrates (lactose), proteins (albumin and others), minerals, and amino acids. BCAA make up 24% of whey protein. No research shows any benefit in healthy people. Some research suggests that whey protein is more effective than casein for promoting muscle mass during weight training. However, soy protein may be as effective as whey protein. Research as to whether whey protein can promote weight loss is ongoing. The best protein source is still real foods because they provide essential nutrients.

Yohimbe

Claims	Enhances energy and stamina.
Other Names	Johimbi, Yohimbine.

Yohimbe

How It Works	Yohimbe may work in several ways, but primarily it works by blocking selected receptors that control the nervous system.
Dose	A dose equivalent to 15–30 mg of Yohimbe daily is typical for impotence. No dose has been established for stamina.
Adverse Effects	Yohimbe may cause high blood pressure, headaches, anxiety, dizziness, and sleeplessness and increase heart rate.
Comments	Yohimbine is derived from the inner bark of an evergreen tree native to Zaire, Cameroon, and Gabon. Yohimbe has been used for centuries as an aphrodisiac, and is used to treat erectile dysfunction. Yohimbe interacts with many other dietary supplements, and should not be used. No data indicate it improves stamina.

Dietary Supplements for Weight Loss

Supplements that may aid in weight loss can be grouped according to how they affect the body. They are typically classified as appetite suppressants, thermogenic agents, or digestion inhibitors. The number of weight loss supplements is staggering. In January 2007, the Federal Trade Commission fined four prominent weight loss supplement (Xenadrine EFX, CortiSlim, Trim Spa, and One-A-Day WeightSmart) manufacturers for deceptive advertising. Many weight loss supplements make claims of effectiveness without reliable scientific evidence. Buyer beware!

Appetite Suppressants

Some dietary supplements marketed as natural appetite suppressants are 5-HTP and Hoodia. Several prescription and over the counter (OTC) medications, such as Wellbutrin, Redux, Meridia, and dexatrin, are also appetite suppressants. More recently, Alli (pronounced ally), whose active ingredient is Orlistat, was approved as the first over-the-counter, FDA-approved weight loss pill. In certain circumstances, Active Duty personnel may be prescribed a weight loss medication for a limited time, under the care of a physician.

5-Hydroxytryptophan or 5-HTP

Claims	Promotes weight and/or body fat loss.
Other Names	5-hydroxy L-tryptophan, 5-Hydroxy Tryptophan, 5-L-Hydroxytryptophan and L-5 HTP.
How It Works	5- HTP crosses the blood brain barrier and increases production of serotonin in the central nervous system. Serotonin can affect sleep, appetite, temperature, and pain sensation.
Dose	A typical dose is 150–300 mg/daily. No dose has been established for weight loss.
Adverse Effects	May cause gastrointestinal symptoms, such as heartburn, stomach pain, flatulence, nausea, vomiting, diarrhea, and loss of appetite. Safety concerns are comparable to tryptophan: 5-HTP has may cause eosinophilia myalgia syndrome (EMS) because of certain contaminants.
Comments	5-HTP or 5-hydroxytryptophan is related to both L-tryptophan and serotonin. In the body, L-tryptophan is converted to 5-HTP, which can then be converted to serotonin.

Hoodia

Claims	Achieve weight or body fat loss.
Other Names	Cactus, Hoodia Gordonii Cactus, Hoodia P57, Kalahari Cactus, Kalahari Diet, P57, Xhoba.
How It Works	Contains a substance that is believed to be an appetite suppressant.
Dose	No established dose has proven effective for weight loss.
Adverse Effects	None yet reported due to lack of published research.

Hoodia

Comments Hoodia gordonii, Hoodia P57 or Kalahari Cactus, is a succulent plant that grows in the Kalahari Desert in southern Africa. It was used by bushman to minimize sensations of hunger.

Other Supplements

Chondroitin Sulfate

Claims Alleviates pain and improves function in persons with osteoarthritis.

Other Names Chondroitin Polysulfate, CPS, CS, CSA, CSC, GAG.

How It Works Chondroitin is found in cartilaginous tissues where it functions to form the joint matrix structure; it may also protect cartilage against degradation by inhibiting a particular enzyme.

Dose A typical dose is 200–400 mg two to three times daily or 1,000–1,200 mg as a single daily dose.

Adverse Effects Chondroitin appears to be well-tolerated, although some people experience can have stomach pain and/or nausea.

Comments Products containing chondroitin or chondroitin plus glucosamine vary greatly in quality and label claims. Make sure the product is USP approved. Chondroitin plus glucosamine combinations that also contain manganese may be the more effective products.

Dehydroepiandrosterone

Claims Dehydroepiandrosterone (DHEA) is used for a multitude of different reasons to include reversing the effects of aging, weight loss, enhancing immune function, increasing strength, energy, and muscle mass, depression, and diabetes.

Dehydroepiandrosterone

Other Names	DHEA
How It Works	DHEA is produced in the adrenal glands, liver, brain and testes of men. DHEA and its sulfate ester, dehydroepiandrosterone sulfate (DHEA-S), act on many tissues, but the actual way it might work is not certain. For sure it has potent actions in the brain, and limited actions as a testosterone promoter.
Dose	The dose depends on the use. Typically 25–50 mg daily are used for the elderly whereas up to 90 mg is used for depression. Up to 200 mg daily has been used.
Adverse Effects	No real adverse effects have been noted at doses below 75 mg daily.
Comments	DHEA can be chemically made or derived from natural sources, such as soy and wild yam. However, these natural sources have no effect on blood levels of DHEA. Natural products (wild yam and soy) labeled, as "natural DHEA" should be avoided. DHEA products have been shown to contain 0%–150% of what is stated on the label. Lastly, DHEA is banned by the National Collegiate Athletic Association.

Fish Oils

Claims	Used to decrease blood lipids, protect against coronary heart disease and high blood pressure; used to decrease inflammation and symptoms of asthma.
Other Names	Cod Liver Oil, Marine Lipid Oil, Marine Oils, Menhaden Oil, N-3 Fatty Acids, N3-polyunsaturated Fatty Acids, Omega 3, Omega-3 Fatty Acids, Omega-3 Marine Triglycerides, Polyunsaturated Fatty Acids (PUFA), Salmon Oil, W-3 Fatty Acids.

Fish Oils

How It Works	Fish oils are high in the omega-3 fatty acids eicosapentaenoic acid (EPA) and docosahexaenoic acid (DHA), which have anti-inflammatory and antithrombotic (preventing aggregation and entrapment of cellular debris) effects.
Dose	Doses range from 1–3 grams/day in a single or two divided doses. Doses over 3 grams are discouraged.
Adverse Effects	Can cause breath and burps to taste and smell like fish. May experience heartburn and/or nausea. Doses greater than 3 grams per day might adversely affect immune function.
Comments	Fish oils come from a variety of marine life including mackerel, herring, sardines, tuna, halibut, salmon, cod liver, and trout. Shellfish, such as oyster, shrimp, and scallop contain less. Evidence is rapidly accumulating that taking fish oil, as food or a supplement, has a very positive impact on health.

Ginkgo Biloba

Claims	Improve memory and concentration; prevent or minimize altitude sickness.
Other Names	Fossil Tree, Ginkgo Folium, Japanese Silver Apricot, Kew Tree, Maidenhair Tree.
How It Works	Ginkgo contains many flavonoids or substances with antioxidant properties. It may work by protecting against free radical damage.
Dose	Doses of 120–600 mg per day have been used for improving memory and 120 mg twice a day for preventing altitude sickness. Doses over 120 mg at any one time may cause mild gastrointestinal problems.
Adverse Effects	Well tolerated but may cause mild gastrointestinal problems, headache, dizziness, and constipation. Increased risk of bleeding.

Ginkgo Biloba

Comments   The Ginkgo tree, also known as the Maidenhair Tree, is unique, and may be the oldest tree in the world. The female tree yields an apricot-like structure containing nuts, fruit or seeds that are eaten for health benefits and for special occasions. The substances from the ginkgo leaf are also extracted for medical uses. Studies regarding its efficacy for altitude sickness are varied—some report success and others no success. Ginkgo may help some and not others, but who will benefit is unknown.

Glucosamine

Claims   Reduces symptoms associated with osteoarthritis, joint pain, back pain, and possibly other musculo-skeletal problems.

Other Names   Glucosamine hydrochloride, glucosamine sulfate and N-Acetyl glucosamine. Chitosamine, D-glucosamine HCl, Glucosamine, Glucosamine HCl, Glucosamine KCl, Glucose-6-Phosphate.

How It Works   Glucosamine hydrochloride is a constituent of cartilage and is required for the formation and maintenance of tendons, ligaments, and cartilage.

Dose   Typical doses are 500 mg three times daily alone or in combination with chondroitin sulfate.

Adverse Effects   Mild gastrointestinal symptoms such as gas, abdominal bloating, and cramps have been reported.

Comments   Glucosamine is usually derived from the outer structure of marine organisms or produced synthetically. Read glucosamine product labels carefully for content. Avoid confusion with glucosamine sulfate and N-acetyl glucosamine because these products may not be interchangeable. Glucosamine sulfate has been studied the most for osteoarthritis. Great variability exists among glucosamine and glucosamine plus chondroitin products. Make sure the product is USP approved. Discuss these products with your physician.

Melatonin

Claims	Acts as a sleep agent; defends against jet lag and oxidant stress.
Other Names	MLT, Pineal Hormone.
How It Works	The hormone, melatonin is produced in the pineal gland and released into the circulation, where it binds to areas in the brain.
Dose	A typical dose for insomnia is 0.3–5.0 mg or 3–5 mg for promoting sleep during transcontinental flights to alleviate jet lag.
Adverse Effects	Minimal to no side effects are noted. Those noted include drowsiness, headache, and dizziness.
Comments	Oral administration of melatonin has a rapid, transient, and mild sleep-inducing effect. Melatonin is also used to advance the body clock before eastward flights by ingesting up to 5 mg in the evening of the days before departure. Melatonin is derived from serotonin (via tryptophan and 5-HTP), which is converted to N-acetylserotonin, and then to melatonin.

Quercetin

Claims	May be a substitute for ibuprofen/motrin/ and other anti-inflammatory agents.
Other Names	Bioflavonoid, Bioflavonoid Complex, Bioflavonoid Concentrate, Bioflavonoid Extract, Citrus Bioflavones, Citrus Bioflavonoid, Citrus Bioflavonoid Extract, Citrus Flavones, Citrus Flavonoids.
How It Works	Acts as an antioxidant and anti-inflammatory agent.
Dose	A typical dose is 400–500 mg three times daily, but 500 mg twice daily has been used. The appropriate dose for anti-inflammatory actions is unclear.

Quercetin

Adverse Effects	May cause headache and tingling of the extremities.
Comments	Quercetin is a flavonoid found in red wine, tea, onions, green tea, apples, berries, broccoli, spinach, cabbage, cauliflower, Brussels sprouts, kale, collard greens, pak choi and kohlrabi. It is also a component of Ginkgo biloba and St. John's Wort. Many forms of quercetin are not well absorbed, which results in low bioavailability.

Tryptophan (L)

Claims	Induces sleep.
Other Names	L-trypt, L-Tryptophan
How It Works	L- tryptophan acts on the brain to induce sleep.
Dose	Doses of 0.3–6 grams per day have been used, with 1–2.5 grams being most common for sleep.
Adverse Effects	L-tryptophan has been linked to eosinophilia myalgia syndrome (EMS) and several deaths; 95% of the cases were traced to a product produced in Japan.
Comments	L-tryptophan may be beneficial as a sleep aid. Dietary tryptophan from protein sources is first converted into 5-HTP (see below) and then to serotonin, which has calming effects. Tryptophan should be obtained from food, such as milk, cheese, meats, poultry, and soy foods. Tryptophan should not be taken in combination with sedating products or herbals, such as 5-HTP, St. John's wort, kava, skullcap, or valerian.

Turmeric

Claims	May have pain-reducing and anti-inflammatory properties. Also used to treat upset stomachs.
Other Names	Curcumin, Indian Saffron, Radix Curcumae, Rhizoma Cucurmae Longae.
How It Works	Appears to inhibit the inflammatory pathways, similar to NSAIDs.
Dose	No dose established for anti-inflammatory actions; 500 mg four times daily has been used for stomach upsets.
Adverse Effects	Tolerated if dose is appropriate; may cause gastrointestinal distress.
Comments	Turmeric is a perennial plant of the ginger family, and native to tropical South Asia. Plants are gathered to obtain the thickened stem (rhizomes) that grows below or on the soil surface. Turmeric is frequently used to flavor or color curry powders, mustards, butters, and cheeses.

Thermogenic Agents

None of these agents should be used.

A multitude of thermogenic or "energy metabolism boosting" substances are available on the market. The most common ingredients in dietary supplements marketed to promote weight loss are bitter orange (Citrus aurantium), country mallow or heartleaf (Sida cordofilia), and ephedra. Others are marketed as "fat burners." Each carries a significant degree of risk, particularly when used during exercise training and extreme environmental conditions, such as a warm environment, diving, and at altitude.

Bitter Orange and Country Mallow

Claims	Increase metabolic rate and induce weight loss.

Bitter Orange and Country Mallow

Other Names	Orange Peel Extract, Seville Orange, Shangzhou Zhiqiao, Sour Orange, Synephrine, Citrus aurantium, and/or Zhi Shi, Heartleaf and White Mallow.
How It Works	Synephrine, like ephedra, is a stimulant that increases heart rate and blood pressure.
Dose	Since serious adverse effects have been linked to low doses of these substances, there is no known safe or recommended dose for these products. The ephedra ban was upheld after a recent court challenge in Feb 2007; the Food and Drug Administration has submitted recommendations to have both bitter orange and country mallow added to the ephedra ban.
Adverse Effects	Bitter orange and country mallow all contain ephedrine or synephrine, which has been linked to serious cardiovascular, or heart, events to include ischemic stroke, rapid heart rate, heart attacks, and even death.
Comments	Manufacturers have substituted synephrine in products that previously contained ephedra. Marketed as ephedra-free, they typically contain synephrine from bitter orange and/or country mallow, plus caffeine and/or caffeine-containing supplements. These may pose the same or greater risks than the original product that contained ephedra. Bitter orange has Generally Recognized as Safe (GRAS) status in the US and is commonly found in foods.

Conjugated Linolenic Acid (CLA)

Claims	Improves body composition/decrease fat mass in overweight or obese persons; reduces hunger.
Other Names	Conjugated LA, CLA-Triacylglycerol, LA, Linoleic Acid.
How It Works	CLA may help shrink fat tissue by inducing cell death of fat cells.

Conjugated Linolenic Acid (CLA)

Dose	Doses ranging from 2–7 grams per day have been used, but more than 3.4 grams per day does not confer additional benefit.
Adverse Effects	CLA has been associated with gastrointestinal distress to include nausea, loose stools, and heart burn. One form of CLA might predispose to type 2 diabetes and cardiovascular disease.
Comments	Although CLA appears to reduce hunger, this is not associated with a reduction in energy intake.

Ephedra

Ephedra has been banned and should not be used under any circumstances.

Garcinia Cambogia or HCA

Claims	Inhibits conversion of excess calories to body fat.
Other Names	Hydroxycitrate, Hydroxycitric Acid, Super Citri-Max, Citrimax, Citrilean, Citrinate and Malabar Tamarinda.
How It Works	Garcinia may interfere with fat production by inhibiting the formation of fatty acids. It may also lower the formation of LDL and triglycerides. In addition, HCA may suppress appetite by promoting glycogen synthesis.
Dose	Several different doses have been used: 300 mg three times daily; 500 mg four times daily; and 1000 mg three times daily. Doses up to 2800 mg/day appear to be safe for short periods of time (up to 90 days).
Adverse Effects	Can cause nausea, gastrointestinal distress and/or headache.
Comments	No conclusive evidence is available that Garcinia cambogia or HCA promotes any significant changes in weight.

Digestion Inhibitors

Digestion inhibitors are typically high fiber products, such as psyllium, chitosan, glucomannan, guar gum, guggul and inulin.

Claims	Prevent weight gain by blocking the absorption or digestion of food.
How It Works	They may slow digestion and interfere with or prevent the absorption of fat and carbohydrates.
Dose	Each product promotes a certain dose. For example, chitosan has been used in doses ranging from 1–5 grams and with other inhibitors. A specific combination of 1.2 grams of chitosan combined with 1.2 grams of glucomannan daily has been used. Also, 2.5 grams of chitosan with 1 gram of psyllium have been used.
Adverse Effects	Major potential problems include gastrointestinal upset, nausea, gas, bulky stools, and constipation.
Comments	Chitosan appears to block the absorption of 5–9 grams of fat daily; which is equivalent to only 45–81 kcal/day. Therefore, these products may not be effective for weight loss.

The Good, the Bad and the Ugly Facts

The following supplements are categorized as "good" due to the availability of data derived from scientific, controlled studies that have demonstrated safety and effectiveness of these products for specific conditions.

The Good Facts

Multivitamins for Protection from "Vending Machine Malnutrition"

A daily multivitamin/mineral supplement providing less than 100% of the RDI for any one nutrient is reasonable for individuals that consistently fail to consume a balanced diet. However, it is important to avoid "mega" dose products that supply 1000% of the RDI for beta-carotene, vitamin A, vitamin E and other fat-soluble vitamins. Long-term use of high doses of fat-soluble vitamins can cause toxicity symptoms.

Chromium

- May be beneficial in lowering blood glucose and blood lipid levels in patients with diabetes.

The Bad Facts

None of the following products should be used.

The following supplements are listed as "bad" due to serious health risks or adverse effects linked to use.

Steroids and Steroid-Enhancers

These agents have been linked to liver toxicity, testicular shrinkage, breast enlargement in males, adverse effects on lipid levels and increased risk of heart attack and stroke.

Andro and Andro precursors

- Banned for use by military personnel!
- Listed as Schedule III controlled substances (cocaine and heroin are also on this list).

Hemp Oil

From the seed of the hemp plant.

- Widely used in body care products, lubricants, paints and industrial uses.
- Hemp oil is deliberately manufactured to contain no significant amounts of THC and is therefore not a psychoactive drug.
- Banned for use by Air Force personnel.
- Pop positive for marijuana on drug urinalysis.

Ephedra (Ephedra sinica)

- Ephedra is a naturally occurring substance derived from botanicals. The principal active ingredient is ephedrine, an amphetamine-like compound that stimulates the nervous system and heart.
- Also known as ma huang, Chinese Ephedra, Ephedrine, Ephedrine Alkaloid, Herbal Ecstasy, Sea Grape, Teamster's Tea, Yellow Astringent, Yellow Horse.
- Ephedra is illegal: On August 17, 2006 the U.S. Court of Appeals for the Tenth Circuit in Denver upheld the FDA final rule declaring all

dietary supplements containing ephedrine alkaloids adulterated, and therefore illegal for marketing in the United States.

- Ephedra can cause life-threatening adverse effects in some people. Multiple case reports have linked ephedra to hypertension, myocardial infarction (MI), seizure, stroke, psychosis, and death.

- Ephedra is a stimulant that can cause heart arrhythmias and cardiac failure.

Synephrine Compounds: Bitter Orange (Citrus aurantium) and Country Mallow, or Heartleaf (Sida cordofolia)

- Present in "ephedra free" compounds but the effects are comparable to ephedra.

- Effects on blood pressure and heart rate are enhanced when taken with caffeine-containing herbals such as guarana, kola nut, mate, green tea and black tea.

No approved thermogenic agents have been shown to be safe and effective for weight loss!

Valerian

- Sold as a sleep aid and does have a sedative effect.

- Mixed with alcohol, it can be dangerous—increases sedative effect.

Kava Kava

- Linked to liver damage and liver failure!

- Banned in European countries and Canada.

St. Johns Wort

- Effective in treatment of mild depression.

- Interferes with a huge number of medications, including birth control pills, blood pressure medication, diabetes and cholesterol medications and anti-depressants.

- Safety warnings now posted in other countries.

5-HTP or 5-Hydroxytryptophan

- Preliminary results indicate that 900 mg/day decrease carbohydrate consumption and causes early satiety and weight loss.

- Serious safety concerns due to cases of EMS (Eosinophilia myalgia syndrome).

Aristolochia

- Used as an aphrodisiac and immune stimulant.

- Contains aristolochic acid, which is nephrotoxic and carcinogenic.

- FDA considers all products containing aristolochic acid to be unsafe and adulterated.

- Although illegal, is still available for sale over the internet.

Usnea or Usnic acid

- Used for weight loss and pain relief.

- A lichen or type of fungus found in a weight loss product called Lipokinetix.

- Linked to liver damage and liver failure.

- Warning issued by FDA on this product.

Salvia

- A perennial herb from the mint family that is native to certain areas of Oaxaca, Mexico.

- Used by the Mazatec Indians for ritual divination and healing.

- Can induce hallucinations, changes in perception, and other psychological effects.

- Can provoke introverted feelings, mild paranoia, excessive sweating and confusion.

- Can induce unconsciousness and short-term memory loss.

- Could seriously undermine military missions.

Herbal formulas with multiple ingredients
are risky because the quantities and
purity are unknown or measured!

The Ugly Facts

Popular products are considered "ugly" if no legitimate scientific research or supporting claim of safety and effectiveness are available or if adverse events are linked to the use of these products. A list of products with on legitimate evidence to support their claims is provided. Buyer beware!

Products with No Legitimate Evidence to Support Claims

Boron	Garcinia Cambogia	Nitric Oxide
Branched Chain AA	Ginkgo Biloba	Pycnogenol
Carnitine	Ginseng	Pyruvate
Chrysin	Glutamine	Taurine
CoEnzyme Q10	Hoodia	Tribulus Terrestris
Conjugated Linoleic Acid	Hydroxycitric Acid/ HCA	Turmeric
Cordyceps	5-Hydroxytryptophan	Whey Protein
DHEA	Lysine	Yohimbe

Energy Drinks

Energy drinks are beverages designed to give a burst of energy. Typically they contain a combination of sugars, caffeine, B vitamins, amino acids, and/or herbal ingredients. The amino acids may include taurine, carnitine, creatine, leucine and the herbals may include guarana (extracts from the guarana plant), ginseng, maltodextrin, and/or ginkgo biloba. Some energy drinks contain inositol and glucuronolactone. The FDA currently does not regulate energy drinks and minimal research has been done on them. The long-term effects of the various energy drink ingredient contaminations are unknown. Most claims are misleading and have not been proven. Potential side effects of energy drinks include an increase in heart rate and blood pressure, anxiety, and nervousness. Energy drinks should not be used while exercising, during training or missions or with alcohol because of the multiple combinations of ingredients, and the possibilities of gastrointestinal distress and disturbances in heart rhythms.

Caffeine is a common ingredient in energy drinks. The caffeine content of energy drinks ranges from 33 mg to nearly 80 mg per serving, with most drinks providing more than the FDA recommended limit for colas. SoBe No Fear had 141 mg in a 16-oz. serving, in contrast to 55 mg, 46 mg, and 37 mg in 12 oz of Mountain Dew, Diet Coke, and Pepsi Cola, respectively.

Taurine is also a common ingredient in energy drinks. The amount of taurine obtained from these beverages is three or more times higher than what is typically obtained through the diet. Limited information from either animal or human studies is available to assess the risk of excessive taurine intake. Also, potential interactions between taurine and caffeine have not been adequately studied.

Glucuronolactone, an ingredient in many energy drinks, occurs naturally in the body when glucose breaks down. The glucuronolactone content of the drinks varies between 2000 mg/L and 2400 mg/L. The daily intake of glucuronolactone from a normal diet is only 1.2 to 2.3 mg and the intake of glucuronolactone from energy drinks is several hundred times higher. The potential effects of excessive glucuronolactone intake are unknown.

Table 2 on the following page presents the amounts of various ingredients in some popular energy drinks.

"The resilience and determination of older operators beats the youthful use of untested supplements."

Warner D. "Rocky" Farr, COLONEL, U.S. ARMY, Command Surgeon, USSOCOM

Beverage, Serving Size	Caffeine (mg)	Taurine (mg)	Ginseng (mg)	Guarana extract (mg)	L-Carnitine (mg)	GRL (mg)*
Red Bull, 8.3 oz	80	1000	–	–	–	600
Monster Energy, 8 oz	70	1000	200	*	*	Unknown amount
Arizona Green Tea, 8 oz	7.5	1000	100	100	–	100
Rockstar Original, 8 oz	80	1000	25	25	25	–
Rockstar Juiced, 8 oz	80	1000	25	25	25	–
Full Throttle, 16 oz	144	605	90	.70	14	–
SoBe No Fear, 8 oz	83	1000	50	50	25	–
SoBe Adrenaline Rush, 8.3 oz	78	1000	25	50	250	–
Amp, 8.4 oz	75	10	10	150	–	–
Crunk Juice, 8.3 oz	100	–	–	–	–	–
Spark, 8 oz	120	200	–	–	10	–
Rush, 8.3 oz	50	1000	–	–	Unknown Amount	1505
Redline, 8 oz	250	–	–	–	–	637
Bookoo, 8 oz	120	1000	–	–	–	–
Socko, 8 oz	80	1000	20	25	–	75

Table 11–2. Supplement Content of Energy Drinks

12 Enemy Agents

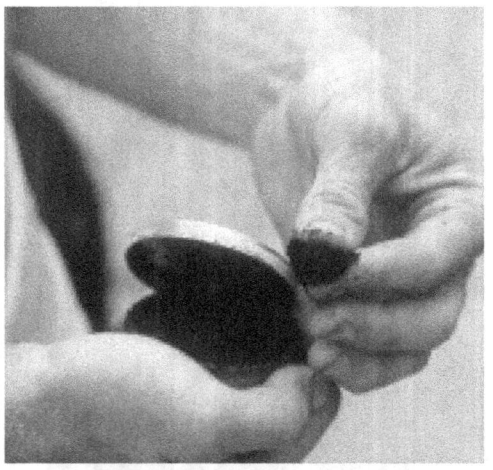

Enemy Agents:
Substances that impair physical,
mental, or psychological performance or compromise health.

Key Points

- All tobacco products, including smokeless tobacco, are addictive, and can cause cardiovascular damage and various forms of cancer.

- Alcohol, in excess, can lead to dehydration and compromise performance. Do not mix drugs and alcohol: beware of alcohol-drug interactions.

- Over-the-counter drugs, such as antihistamines, non-steroidal anti-inflammatory drugs, and aspirin should be used in moderation and under a physician's care if being used for long-term therapy.

- NSAIDs should not be used during deployments because they make bleeding difficult to control.

- Steroids and steroid alternatives are illegal and unsafe; they can seriously harm the body and negatively affect performance.

Enemy agents are substances that may pose significant detrimental effects on health, even if some may enhance performance or make one feel better, be it physical, mental, or psychological. If these agents are used, it is important to be aware of their potential harmful effects, on either health or performance. The enemy agents of interest in this chapter will be chewing tobacco, alcohol, antihistamines, steroids, non-steroidal anti-inflammatory medications, other over-the-counter products, and ephedra.

Smokeless Tobacco (ST)

Like 7.3 million persons in the United States, many military personnel have been or are frequent users of smokeless tobacco (ST). The majority of people who use ST are young and middle age adult males. The primary reason ST is considered an enemy agent is because of its adverse effects on health. Persons who use ST have:

- 50-fold higher risk of oral cancer than those who do not use ST.

- Increased risk for gum disease.

- Permanent tooth stains.

- Bad breath.

- Sores on the lips and mouth.

- Tooth decay, because of the sugar added to ST.

- Increased blood pressure and heart rate.

- Increased levels of LDL cholesterol, the "bad" cholesterol.

One reason the risk of cancer is so high is because ST products contain at least 28 chemicals that may cause cancer. Despite these issues, many athletes and Warfighters believe that ST improves performance or enhances reaction time by providing a quick "rush" during the event, but this is usually not the case.

Nicotine

Nicotine, the active ingredient in all tobacco products, is very addicting (as addicting as cocaine or heroin), and nicotine addiction is one of the most prevalent addictive behaviors worldwide. Nicotine is a naturally occurring "alkaloid," like caffeine, that exerts potent effects on the human body. It is considered a psychoactive drug, which means it alters the normal functioning of the brain by stimulating the central nervous system. This results in the nicotine "buzz," or "high." When ST is placed in the mouth, the nicotine is readily taken up into the small blood vessels that line the mouth and gums, after which it travels through the bloodstream to the brain where it exerts multiple effects.

Nicotine initially causes a rapid release of adrenaline, the "fight-or-flight" hormone, which increases heart rate, blood pressure, and blood glucose. However, the results of nicotine's effects are short-lived and may last only 40 minutes to a couple of hours. After a period of time the effects of nicotine are lessened, and more and more nicotine is needed to achieve the same degree of stimulation or relaxation.

Although nicotine and tobacco have enough disadvantages to discourage their use, it is important to remember that, in certain situations, they may provide desirable effects. This is why leaders, like George Washington during the Revolutionary War, request "necessary" items like food, munitions, and tobacco for their troops. The reported "benefits" of nicotine include:

- Decreased appetite.

- Control of or reduction in body weight.

- Ability to focus attention.

- Increased energy.

- Decreased pain.

The ability to focus attention or "enhance mental state" is why users claim their reaction time and performance are enhanced. However, no studies have shown differences in reaction times between users and non-users of smokeless tobacco. Remember: there are **no** reaction time improvements with chew.

Nicotine has some very detrimental effects. It:

- Increases blood pressure, heart rate, and rate of respiration.

- Constricts/tightens blood vessels, which is why increases in blood pressure and heart rate are seen. One study of young athletes showed that the amount of blood the heart pumped in one minute decreased while using ST. This would be highly undesirable for Warfighters during strenuous exercise, and could compromise performance particularly in a warm environment.

- Stimulates the nervous system.

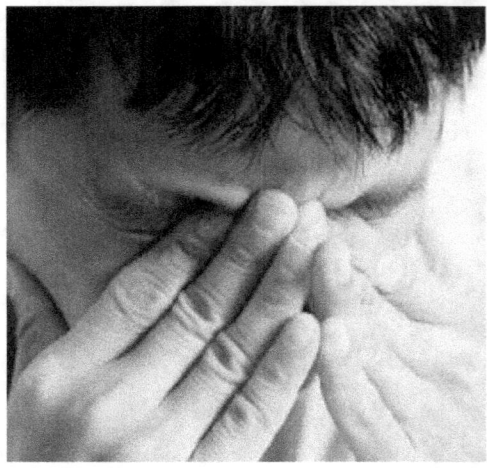

Nicotine Withdrawal

Repeated or chronic administration of nicotine usually results in drug dependence. Therefore, cessation of nicotine after dependence develops may result in withdrawal effects (see below). Most of these effects last weeks, but some (body weight gain and nicotine craving) may persist a year after cessation.

The adaptations of nicotine dependence may include increasing or decreasing the number of receptors in the brain and/or increasing or decreasing the release of neurotransmitters that signal the brain. The end result is a disturbance in function. Some of the symptoms of trying to quit nicotine include:

The risks of using ST outweigh the benefits.

- Irritability.

- Anxiety.

- Depression.

- Moodiness.

- Headaches.

- Trouble sleeping.

- Poor concentration.

- Craving for nicotine.

- Increased body weight.

The military has many programs for individuals trying to quit smoking and chewing, but it is best to never start.

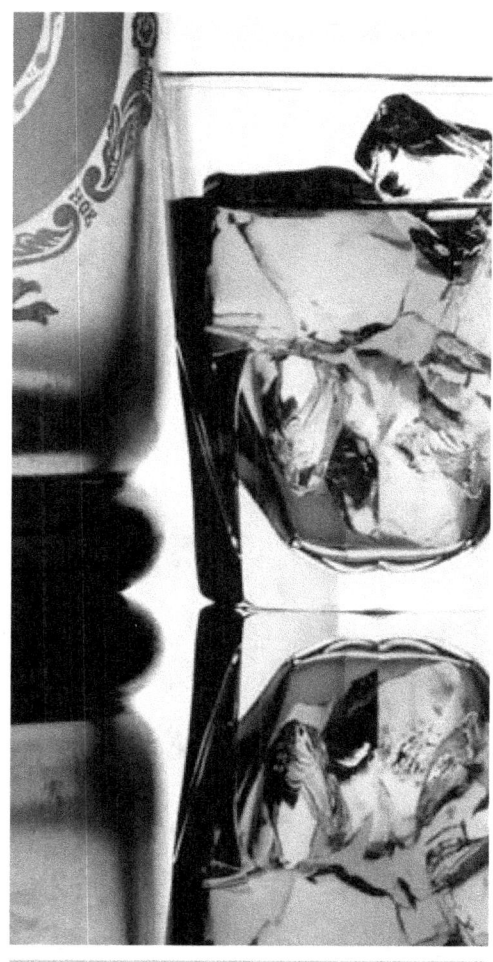

Alcohol

Heavy drinking is a major cause of preventable death. It can damage the liver, heart, and skeletal muscles; increase the chance of developing some cancers, contribute to violence, and interfere with relationships. Individual reactions to alcohol differ, depending on many factors. Important factors include:

- Age.
- Gender.
- Race or ethnicity.
- Genetics.
- Weight.
- Fitness level.
- Amount of food eaten before drinking.
- How quickly alcohol was consumed.
- Use of drugs/prescription medicines.
- Family history of alcohol problems.

Regardless of the factors, alcohol has only negative effects on performance. In particular, drinking alcohol leads to a state of dehydration, in the absence of adequate fluid replacement. People have died during road races and regular training after a night of heavy drinking, due to inadequate rehydration prior to, and hydration during, exercise. Although a rare occurrence, it can happen. More frequently, a dehydrated state places an athlete at greater risk for musculoskeletal injuries (cramps, muscle pulls, and muscle strains), which will clearly compromise mission objectives.

Excessive alcohol intake can lead to severe dehydration.

Alcohol consumption also decreases the use of glucose and amino acics by skeletal muscles, which adversely affects energy supply and metabolic processes during exercise. Chronic alcohol consumption may lead to structural changes in skeletal muscle and a decrease in the size of all muscle fiber types, both of which will adversely affect performance. Alcohol also hinders the muscle's ability to replenish energy stores, which may increase recovery time or compromise rehab after an injury. In addition, athletes who use alcohol have twice the injury rate as non-alcohol users.

In addition to performance decrements, using specific drugs with alcohol can have serious medical consequences. The National Institute on Alcohol

Abuse and Alcoholism (NIAAA) has a publication "Harmful Interactions: Mixing Alcohol with Medicines" that details all of the known interactions. Examples include the increased risk of bleeding in the stomach when aspirin and non-steroidal anti-inflammatory medications are combined. Also, taking medications that contain acetaminophen when drinking beer can greatly increase the risk of liver toxicity. Combining beer with antihistamines, barbiturates (Nembutal, Luminal, Seconal), benzodiazepines (Ativan, Valium, Restoril) and tricyclic antidepressants (Elavil, Pamelor), and other agents used as sleeping aids may increase the sedative effect of these drugs and cause other adverse effects.

Mixing alcohol with drugs can be dangerous!

Antihistamines

Antihistamine use is prevalent among all groups of people because they are common over-the-counter and prescription medications. Many types of antihistamines are used, with the most common "sedating" ones being:

- Diphenhydramine (Benadryl).

- Chlorpheniramine (Chlor-Trimeton).

- Cyproheptadine (Periactin).

- Hydroxyzine (Atarax, Vistaril).

Some detrimental performance and side effects of sedating antihistamines include:

- Decreased ability to concentrate.

- Delayed reaction time.

- Sleepiness.

- More "misses" on target practice.

- Dry mouth.

- Increased heart rate.

- Blurred vision.

- Constipation.

Antihistamines may cause drowsiness and compromise mental performance.

Because of the problem of drowsiness, other "non-sedating" or less sedating types of antihistamines have been developed. The "non" sedating antihistamines include:

- Cetirizine (Zyrtec).

- Fexofenadine (Allegra).

- Loratadine (Claritin).

Allegra (Fexofenadine) is the least sedating, and although Claritin and other Loratadine-containing products are minimally sedating, sedation may occur at higher doses. The antihistamine, Zyrtec (Cetirizine) is considered less sedating than Benadryl, but it can be sedating at the usual dose, so pay attention to individual reactions. No clearly defined effects on physical performance have been reported, but caution should be exercised when taking any type of medication.

The use of anti-histamines, specifically benadryl, has been associated with heat casualties and heat stroke during training. Ranger school has had at least one fatality due to heat stroke in a student who was taking benadryl to treat poison ivy.

NSAID/Vitamin M delays and hampers healing in muscles, ligaments, tendons, and cartilage.

Non-Steroidal Anti-Inflammatory Drugs (NSAIDs)

A number of over-the-counter (OTC) medications, including aspirin and ibuprofen (non-steroidal anti-inflammatory drugs, or NSAIDs) are readily available and widely used by Warfighters, who call these medications "Vitamin M." Vitamin M refers to "Motrin." These drugs are found in most medicine cabinets and in a medic's pack to treat pain, reduce fever, and/or inflammation. However, several dangers are associated with using these medications on a regular basis. They include:

- Potential decrease in the effectiveness of daily aspirin use, if taken at same time as the NSAID.

- Contribute to gastrointestinal problems, including bleeding and ulcers.

- Trigger an asthmatic attack in persons with exercise-induced asthma.

- Mask signs of a more serious medical problem that may require medical intervention.

- Contribute to development of hyponatremia in endurance athletes.

- Cause serious performance and health decrements of some endurance athletes.

- Slow down the healing of muscles, cartilage, ligaments and tendons.

The FDA has requested that package inserts for all NSAIDs include a warning about the potential increased risk of cardiovascular events and, serious, and potentially life-threatening, gastrointestinal bleeding. The clear message is that NSAIDS or Vitamin M should be used on a limited basis. Products with fewer side effects should be used, whenever possible (See Quercitin in Chapter 11). When pain is prolonged or seems to be worsening, medical attention must be sought for a proper evaluation.

With respect to hyponatremia and long distance events, NSAIDs should not be used until after exercise and even then, taken in moderation. A proper warm-up and sound nutritional practices will do more to prevent muscle soreness and inflammation than popping Vitamin M.

Importantly, the mission must be considered before taking NSAIDs as they interfere with clotting. If injured, the use of NSAIDs makes bleeding difficult to control. For general aches and pains, acetaminophen is an alternative. If an NSAID is essential, meloxicam (Mobic) or celecoxib (Celebrex) are alternatives.

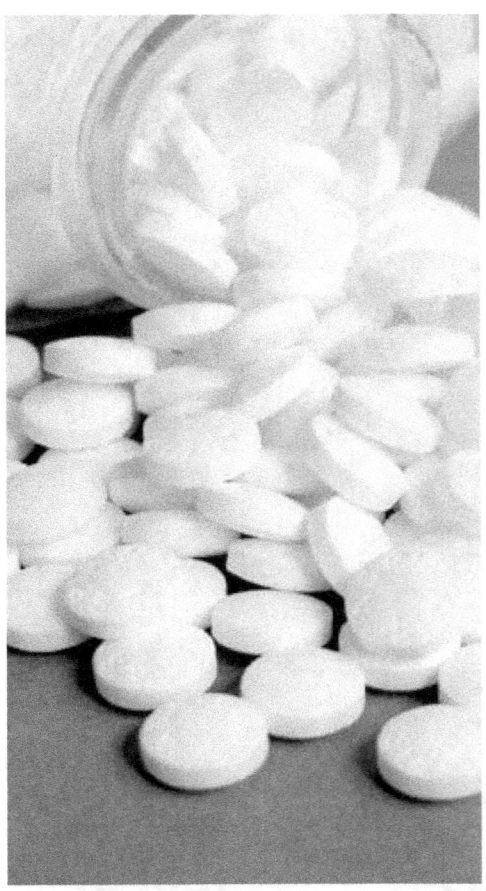

Consult with a physician or pharmacist
prior to using NSAIDS.

Generic Name	Brand Names
Aspirin	Made by several companies
Ibuprofen	Motrin®, Advil®, Motrin IB®
Naproxen	Naprosyn®, Aleve®
Meloxicam	Mobic®

Steroids (Anabolic-Androgenic)

Anabolic steroids are compounds "designed" to behave like testosterone, the primary androgenic or "masculinizing" hormone that builds muscle and enhances male attributes. These steroids are classified as "Controlled Substances" and regulated by the Drug Enforcement Administration (DEA). They are banned by most athletic associations.

Congress passed the Anabolic Steroid Control Act of 2004 in response to a rise in steroid abuse by athletes, teenagers, and, especially, youngsters. This Act redefined the term "anabolic steroid" to mean "any drug or hormonal substance, chemically and pharmacologically related to testosterone (other than estrogens, progestins, corticosteroids, and dehydroepiandrosterone)." Androstenedione, androstenediol, androstanediol, androstanedione and similar substances (total of 26 androgenic and pre-cursor substances) were banned by the FDA in January 2005. Many of these substances, once sold as dietary supplements, became controlled, which means they are in the same category as cocaine and heroin: they are illegal to purchase or use.

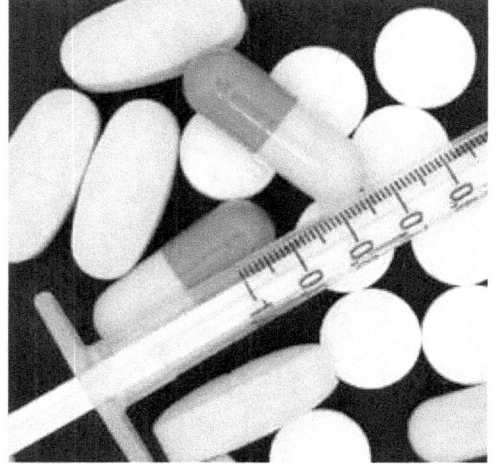

It is important to understand that testosterone itself is not effective when taken orally or by injection because of its rapid degradation by the liver. This is why so many modifications are made to the chemical structure of testosterone with the expectation of finding a substance with actions similar to testosterone. This is the reason why transdermal patches, buccal tablets and nasal sprays are being used as delivery modalities.

Anabolic Steroids and Cycling

Steroids are used illegally by athletes and others to enhance performance and/or improve physical appearance. The use of anabolic-androgenic steroids has been shown to increase body mass, lean body mass, strength, and power, and decrease body fat, which may directly or indirectly enhance performance. Because of these effects, Warfighters may be using them intentionally or unintentionally.

Doses taken by users/abusers may be 10–100 times higher than doses typically used for medical conditions. Anabolic steroids are taken orally or injected, typically in cycles of weeks or months. "Cycling" is when multiple dosages are taken over a period of time and then stopped for a specific period of time before beginning the cycle over again. The primary reason for cycling is to reduce the risk of side effects, which increases with length of time on the drugs.

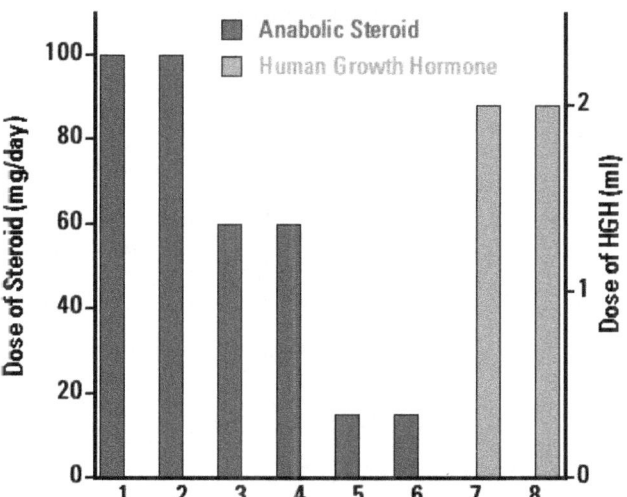

Steroid use will harm the body, both short term and in the long run.

"Stacking" is a method commonly used by steroid (ab)users. Two or more types of steroids may be taken at the same time, sometimes mixing oral and injection drugs. Some drugs may be obtained "off the economy" of a foreign country, or they may be meant for veterinary use. This is a serious concern, because such drugs may be adulterated with other dangerous substances.

"Pyramiding" is another dangerous method of steroid use/abuse. There are many paradigms, but in one case, the person increases the frequency, dosage, and/or adds various types of steroids, followed by decreasing dose and frequency until no drugs are taken. The cycle during "pyramiding" is usually 6–12 weeks, with return to a low/no dose at the end of the cycle. The expected or intended benefits of "cycling," "stacking," and "pyramiding" have not been substantiated scientifically. An example of a "Ski Slope Pyramid" is shown below.

Adverse Effects of Steroids

The well-documented short- and long-term negative side effects of anabolic steroids must be understood. It is very clear that the benefits of performance enhancements and increasing physical attributes do not outweigh the risks involved.

The physical side effects of using steroids are shown in Table 1. However, many behavioral changes occur and may include aggression, violence, irritability, anxiety, distractibility, and abrupt shifts in mood: anabolic steroid users are often vulnerable to depression or rage. Of note is the fact that using anabolic steroids disturbs the regular production of testosterone, which may persist for months after discontinuing the drug. An unknown portion of those who use steroids become addicted to them.

Anabolic steroids should be avoided.

Table 12–1. Possible Health Risks/Consequences of Anabolic Steroid Use		
Hormonal System	**Cardiovascular System**	**Liver**
Shrinking testicles	Increase in LDL (bad cholesterol)/ Decrease in HDL (good cholesterol)	Cancer (Breast, prostrate, pancreatic)
Develop Breasts	High blood pressure	Tumor(s)
Infertility	Heart attack	
Male-pattern baldness	Enlargement of heart's left ventricle	
Skin	**Infection**	**Psychiatric**
Severe acne	HIV/AIDS	Mania
Fluid retention	Hepatitis	Delusions
Oily scalp		Rage
Jaundice		Aggressive Behavior

Stacking

Of great concern is the use of multiple compounds in combination with steroids to counteract the common adverse effects. Other drugs often used with anabolic steroids include diuretics, anti-estrogens, human chorionic gonadotrophin, human growth hormone, thyroid hormone, insulin, gonadotrophin-releasing hormone, clenbuterol, and clomid. This "polypharmacy" practice is a deadly combination, and has resulted in the death of military members.

Agents Recently Banned

Androstenediol

Claims	Enhances recovery and promotes muscle growth from exercise.
Other Names	4-AD, 4-Androstenediol, 5-AD, 5-Androstenediol, Androdiol.
How It Works	A weak steroid hormone and is a direct precursor of testosterone.
Dose	A dose of 100 mg twice daily has been used.
Adverse Effects	At low doses nothing of note. May increase endogenous testosterone production and increase levels of estrone and estradiol.
Comments	Androstenediol does not appear to increase muscle strength or mass when used during 12 weeks of high-intensity resistance training. The Anabolic Steroid Control Act of 2004 reclassified androstenediol from a dietary supplement to an anabolic steroid, a controlled substance.

Androstenedione

Claims	Enhances recovery and promotes muscle growth from exercise.
Other Names	Andro, Androstene.

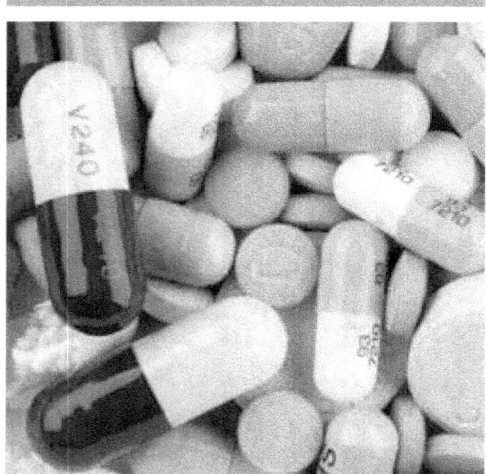
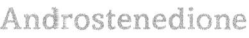

Androstenedione

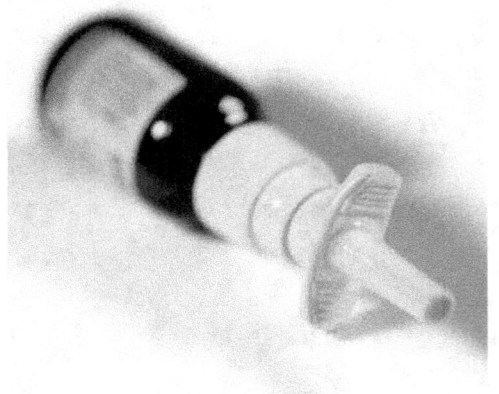

How It Works	A direct precursor of testosterone.
Dose	Doses of 100–300 mg daily have been used without success.
Adverse Effects	May decrease endogenous testosterone production and increase estrogen. Stimulate growth of prostate cancer cells. May increase risk of heart disease in men.
Comments	Taking androstenedione orally in doses of 100-300 mg per day did not result in increased muscle strength or size, or lean body mass when used for 2-3 months during weight training. The Anabolic Steroid Control Act of 2004 reclassified androstenedione from a dietary supplement to an anabolic steroid, a controlled substance.

Multi-Ingredient Steroid Alternatives—The Bottom Line

The increased search for the creation, manufacture, and promotion of new "designer steroids," "pro-steroids," "pro-hormones," and/or "precursor steroids" as over-the-counter anabolic compounds is staggering. Multiple steroid alternative products have surfaced on the market in alarming numbers, but the questions are, do they work, and how well do they work?

Some supplements containing herbs, glandulars, minerals such as chromium and boron, and a number of other compounds (ZMA) are being marketed to build big muscles. They claim to be "alternatives to steroids." The major concerns associated with using such products are:

- Not properly tested and absolutely no basis to substantiate claims.

- Potential for harmful side effects, allergic reactions and toxicities.

- Metabolic pathways and waste products from some compounds are unknown.

- Potential for testing positive for banned substances.

- Expensive and unlikely to replace the benefits of a good diet and sound training program.

Approximately one in five dietary supplements (20%) sold for building muscle and improving athletic performance were contaminated with "steroid-like" chemicals.

Contamination and Adulteration

A large number of "non-hormonal" dietary supplements, like vitamins, minerals, and amino acids, commonly used by athletes and others, are contaminated with and contain prohormones and/or precursor steroids. In 2003 the International Olympic Committee issued a warning of widespread contamination in numerous dietary supplements sold to athletes. These contaminated products included:

- Protein powders and amino acids supplements.
- Creatine.
- Hydroxy-Methyl-Butyrate (HMB).
- Carnitine, ribose, pyruvate.
- Guarana.
- Tribulus Terrestris.
- Vitamins supplements and some mineral supplements containing zinc.
- Numerous herbal extracts.
- Supplements marketed as "pro-hormones" of testosterone.

Ephedra

Ephedra (ma huang), which was discussed in Chapter 11, is an herb containing several substances called ephedra alkaloids (ephedrine and pseudoephedrine). Ephedra was an ingredient in dietary supplements for a number of years until multiple adverse events (heart attack, stroke, and death) were reported. Based on these multiple adverse events, in 2004 the FDA concluded that dietary supplements containing ephedrine alkaloids pose a risk of serious adverse events (heart attack, stroke, and death), and that these risks are unreasonable in light of any benefits that may result from the use of these products. Thus, ephedra became illegal.

FDA has the authority to take action against a dietary supplement when the product (1) presents a significant risk, an unreasonable risk, or an imminent hazard; (2) does not comply with good manufacturing practices, or (3) makes an unsubstantiated structure-function claim. The FDA ruling that banned dietary supplements containing ephedrine alkaloids will remain in effect until further notice. Although it is still available over the internet and some companies are still selling it, this should not be happening. **No product containing ephedra should be purchased or used.**

If a product sounds too good to be true, it is usually not worth trying.

13 Combat Rations

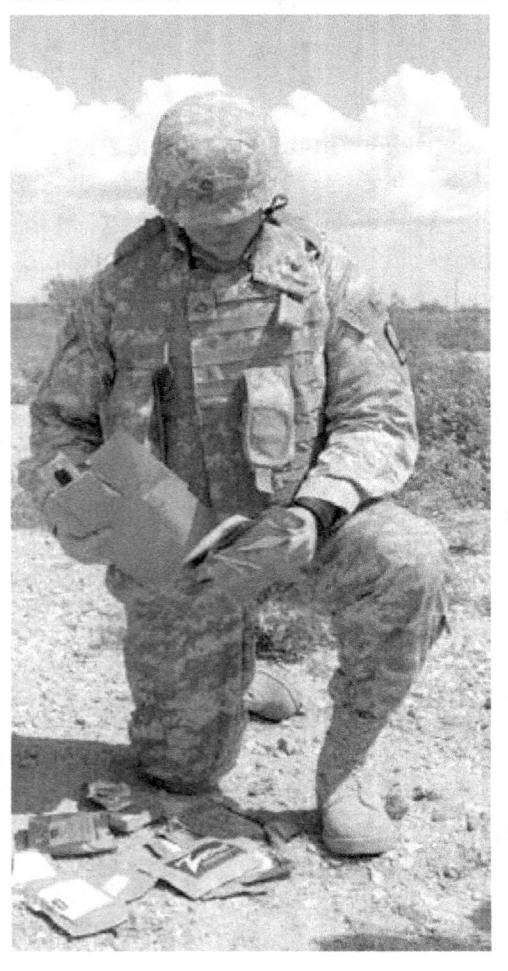

Key Points

- Combat rations are specially designed to supply adequate energy and nutrients for particular types of missions.

- Environmental and operational dictate changes in combat rations to meet nutritional needs.

- Rations provide different amounts of energy to meet the needs of various operational conditions.

- Some rations have been designed to meet strict religious diets.

- Commercial products are available to supplement military rations and/or allow for greater diversity and choice for eating when deployed.

Military rations are the cornerstone of combat and field feeding. Currently, four types of rations are available: Group Feeding, Individually Packaged, Restricted, and Specialty Rations. The type of ration a Warfighter needs depends on the unit's mission, location, and availability of personnel and equipment for preparing meals. All military rations, except the Restricted Rations, are nutritionally adequate, which means they meet the regulations for what a ration must contain. In this chapter an overview and descriptions of selected rations are provided.

The Meal, Ready-to-Eat Individual (MRE) Menus

The **Meal, Ready-to-Eat** (MRE) is designed to sustain an individual engaged in heavy activity when normal food service facilities are not available. The MRE may be consumed as the sole ration for up to 21 days. After 21 days, other appropriate rations should be included. When the MRE is the sole ration, supplements and enhancements (for example, bread, milk, and fresh fruit) should be provided, whenever feasible.

The MRE is a self-contained combat ration. Except for the beverages, the entire meal is ready to eat: rehydration of MREs is not necessary. One MRE packet provides an average of 1,250 kcal with approximately 13% of

Each MRE menu provides an average of 1,250 kcal (13% of energy from protein, 36% from fat, and 51% from CHO).

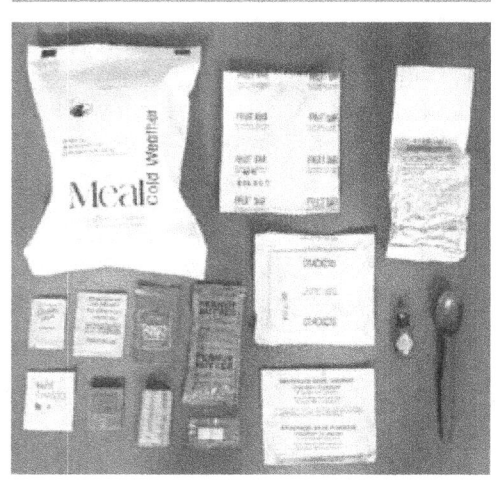

Based on activity level, 2–4 MREs would be needed each day.

energy from protein, 36% from fat, and 51% from CHO: one MRE provides $\frac{1}{3}$ of the Military Recommended Daily Allowance for vitamins and minerals, as deemed essential by the U.S. Surgeon General. Although nutritionally balanced (if all components are eaten), the percentage of energy from fat is higher than current recommendations in the U.S.

Because the different meal components of the MRE are fortified with selected vitamins and minerals, at least some of the contents from each food item must be eaten.

The shelf stable, split-top bread, used to supplement the meal, provides 200 kcals (55% CHO, 12% protein, 33% fat) per pouch.

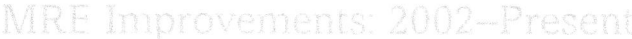

MRE Improvements: 2002–Present

Feedback from Operation Desert Shield/Storm suggested that Warfighters would consume more of the MRE if their preferences were considered. Based on that feedback, the Fielded Individual Ration Improvement Program was initiated to boost up variety, acceptability, palatability, and nutrient distribution of individual combat rations to enhance consumption, and hence, performance, on the battlefield.

The Meal, Cold Weather/Food Packet, Long-Range Patrol (MCW/LRP)

The MCW/LRP serves as an operational ration for two separate scenarios. The **Meal, Cold Weather** (MCW) is intended for cold weather feeding: it will not freeze and extra drink mixes for countering dehydration during cold weather activities are included. Three per day should be issued for a complete cold weather ration. The MCW is packaged in a white camouflage pouch similar to the former Ration, Cold Weather (RCW).

The **Food Packet, Long Range Patrol** (LRP) is a restricted calorie ration meant for missions where resupply is not available and weight and volume are critical factors. One per day is issued to a Warfighter for up to ten days. The LRP is packaged in a tan camouflage menu pouch similar to the current MRE. The menus contain dehydrated entree items, as well as other accessory items.

One menu bag per day is used for the LRP, whereas three menu bags are used per day for MCW. Thus, the MCW provides 4,500 kcal, which is needed to replenish glycogen from exertion in extreme cold. The individual prepares the menu bags, which require 34 ounces of water to hydrate all components in the individual menu bag.

Light Weight Rations

Survival, General Purpose, Improved (GP-I)

The **Food Packet, Survival, General Purpose, Improved** is a restricted ration used to sustain an individual in survival situations (including escape and evasion, under all environmental conditions, and when potable water is limited, for periods of less than 5 consecutive days). The ration contains six compressed bars: 2 cereal bars, 3 cookie bars, and 1 sucrose bar. Lemon tea, sugar, soup, and gravy base are also included. Each packet provides 1,447 kcal (5% protein, 39% fat, and 56% carbohydrate). This ration is designed to provide a maximum of 8% of the energy from protein to minimize metabolic water requirements. The percentage of kcal from fat is higher than typically recommended in order to increase the energy content and minimize total weight: one packet weighs 11.4 ounces. Fourteen ounces of water are required to reconstitute the lemon tea, soup, and gravy base.

Survival, Abandon Ship

The **Food Packet, Survival, Abandon Ship** is used by the Navy to sustain one person for three days (using two bars/day) who must abandon ship; it is designed to fit in the storage areas of lifesaving craft. The packet contains a minimum of six individually wrapped cereal bars. The ration is strictly a short-term survival food to minimize the negative effects of acute starvation. Each packet provides approximately 2,400 kilocalories (54% carbohydrate). The components are compatible with potable water restrictions. No preparation is necessary, except opening packages. The ration weighs 5.2 ounces.

Survival, Aircraft, Life Raft

The **Food Packet, Survival, Aircraft, Life Raft** is used by the Navy to sustain personnel who survive aircraft disasters. The packet, along with other essential equipment, is supplied in emergency kits on naval aircraft. The ration weighs 3.5 ounces and contains hard candy, candy-coated chewing gum, and twine. An instruction sheet explains the use of the twine for storing components after the packet is opened. Each packet provides approximately 300 kcal (100% carbohydrate). It is strictly short-term survival food to minimize the negative effects of acute starvation. The components are compatible with potable water restrictions. No preparation is necessary, except opening packages.

Each menu provides about 1,540 kcals (15% protein, 35% fat, and 50% carbohydrate).

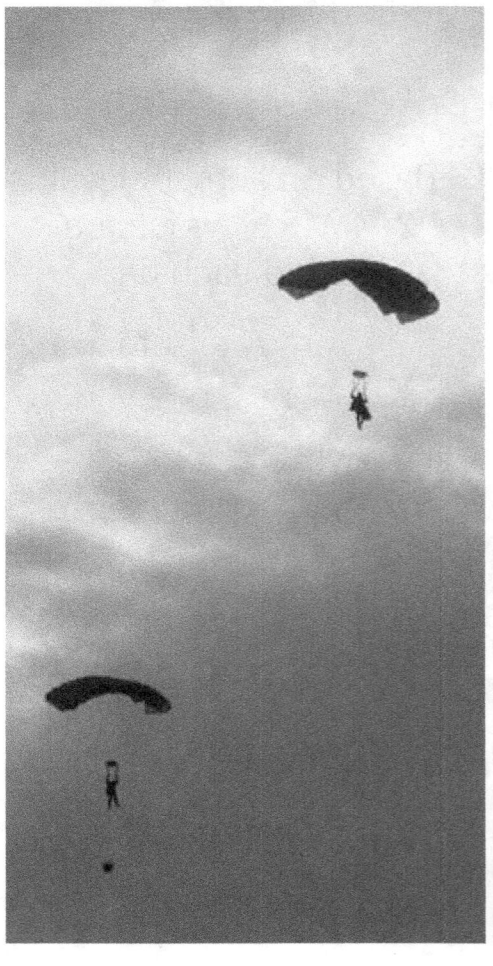

Tailored Operational Training Meal (TOTM)

The **Tailored Operational Training Meal** ration provides an alternative operational training meal in lieu of "sack lunches" and catered commercial meals to organizations that engage in "inactive duty training" (IDT) where traditional operational rations are not mandated. The "train as you fight" philosophy is being promoted. Using this meal during training will allow units to become familiar with pre-packed meals, similar to MRE. The TOTM is similar to the standard MRE in packaging and contains many of the same components. However, it employs commercial packaging to reduce costs.

The TOTM is not an MRE, nor is it designed to take the place of the MRE. It is a lightweight, totally self-contained packet consisting of a meal in a flexible meal bag that fits easily into military field clothing pockets. A TOTM typically contain an entrée, wet-pack fruit, a beverage base, flameless heater, dining kit, and other assorted components.

The content of one TOTM meal bag
provides an average of 997 kcals.

Except for the beverages, the entire meal is ready to eat. The entree may be eaten cold when operationally necessary, but it can also be heated in a variety of ways, including immersion in hot water. A flameless heating device is included in each meal bag to heat the entree.

Meal, Religious, Kosher/Halal

The **Meal, Religious, Kosher or Halal** is used to feed individuals who maintain a strict religious diet. Each meal consists of one Kosher or Halal certified entree and religiously certified/acceptable complementary items to meet the MDRA. Like the MRE, it is a totally self-contained meal with one entree, plus a bag containing other components.

Each Religious Meal provides approximately
1,200 kcals (11-13% protein, 37-40%
fat, and 48% carbohydrate).

First Strike Rations

Negative energy balance (weight loss) is expected during strenuous sustained operations (SUSOPS). However, the potential accompanying fatigue and mental impairments (confusion, depression, and loss of awareness) can be overcome by appropriate nutrition. The **First Strike Ration**, or FSR, is designed to help sustain physical performance, postpone fatigue and minimize other adverse health consequences experienced during SUSOPS.

The FSR is a compact, eat-on-the-move assault ration designed to be consumed during the first 72 hours of intense conflict by forward deployed Warfighters. The FSR is lightweight and designed to sustain needs during highly mobile, intense operations. All components of this lightweight ration are familiar, eat-out-of-hand foods that require little or no preparation. The beverages must be reconstituted and consumed directly from the drink pouch.

The FSR provides about 2,900 calories, whereas one MRE provides approximately 1,250 calories; it also weighs much less than one MRE. The FSR is not intended for non-combat operations or field training exercises and is not nutritionally complete. The FSR was first delivered to the Warfighters in 2007, and is under revision, as the product provides too much fat and not enough CHO and protein for sustained missions.

Other Rations and Ration Components

Unitized Group Rations—A (UGR-A) Menu Improvements

The most efficient way to get breakfast, lunch and dinner to large groups of Warfighters around the world is the **Unitized Group Ration**. The 50 complete meals are packed together in the UGR. They have been improved over the past few years.

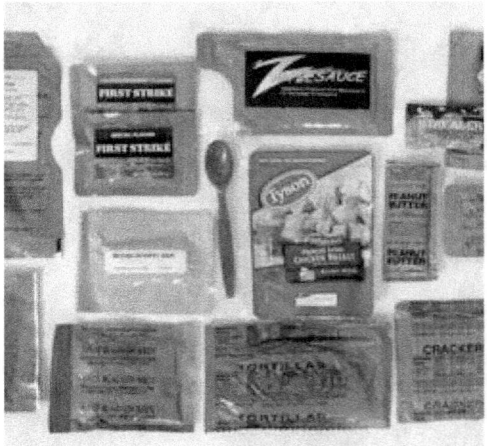

Unitized Group Ration—Express (UGR-E)

The UGR-E is a compact, self-contained module that provides a complete, hot meal for 18 Warfighters. By simply pulling a tab, the food is heated in just 30-45 minutes, and served in trays to Warfighters like a cook prepared meal.

Shelf Stable Pocket Sandwich

Shelf stable pocket sandwiches will enhance the variety of individual ration components while providing a much needed eat-on-the-move capability. Current varieties include Barbecue Beef, Pepperoni, Italian, and Barbecue Chicken—all of which were given high marks during field tests. A Bacon Cheddar

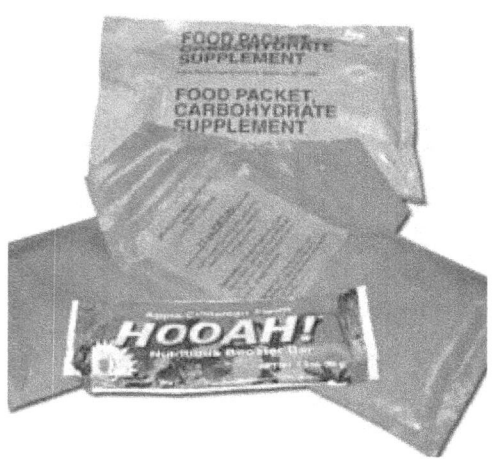

pocket was recently developed to provide a breakfast option and further increase variety. Additional breakfast sandwiches are under development.

Performance Enhancing Ration Components

Carbohydrates, caffeine, vitamins, and antioxidants are some of the food enhancers used to make **Performance Enhancing Ration Components** (PERC). PERCs are formulated to improve the physical and mental performance of Warfighters during sustained operations and under all climatic conditions.

- **Food Packet, Carbohydrate Supplement (CarboPack)**

The **CarboPack** is a ration supplement that provides additional energy to the Warfighter during intense, prolonged physical activity and highly stressful conditions. It consists of two 12 oz carbohydrate electrolyte beverages and one carbohydrate rich bar. It provides a minimum of 75 grams of carbohydrate, four grams of protein, and 380 kilocalories.

- **ERGO Drink**

ERGO stands for **Energy Rich, Glucose Optimized.** This drink is a primary source of carbohydrates (12%) to restore glycogen and speed recovery.

- **HooAH!® Bar**

The bar is formulated for glucose release, but its solid structure means digestion occurs over a longer period of time. The HooAH!© bar helps delay fatigue and extend endurance.

- **Soldier Fuel**

This energy booster gel provides Warfighters an alternative to solid bars for performance enhancement. Laboratory data have shown these products to be effective in maintaining blood glucose, which should provide sustained energy.

- **Next Generation HooAH!® Bar**

These multi-component bars will incorporate selected proteins to conserve lean body mass, probiotics/prebiotics to maintain gastrointestinal integrity, and functionally stable micro/macronutrients to mitigate performance degradation and increase ration consumption.

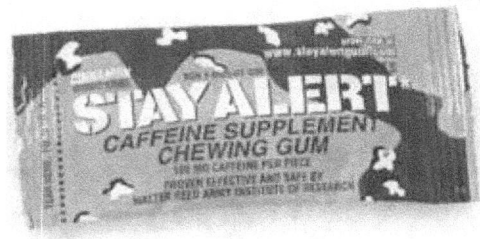

- **Caffeine Gum**

In 2006 the Army introduced "Stay Alert," a caffeinated chewing gum, as a countermeasure for fatigue. Each piece of Stay Alert contains 100 mg of caffeine, which is comparable to a 6 oz cup of coffee. Caffeine is delivered approximately four to five times faster than a liquid, because it is absorbed in the mouth. Stay Alert, also a component of First Strike Rations, is available through military supply channels.

Composition of Rations for Combat Operations

In 2006 a panel of experts (Institute of Medicine) met to examine the energy, carbohydrate, protein, vitamin, and mineral requirements for rations designed to support personnel during short term, high-intensity combat operations. In the end, the requirements were primarily based on DRIs (See Chapter 4), but modifications were made based on sweat losses and nutrient utilization under conditions of high energy expenditure and stress. These requirements were established to help develop the First Strike Ration, and are being used for further ration development.

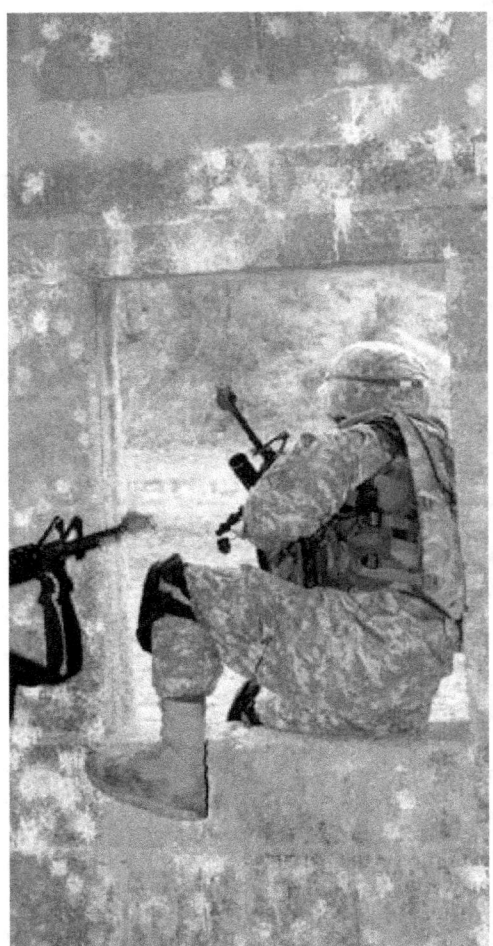

Commercial Freeze-Dried Products

Light weight, freeze-dried foods are commercially available from a number of manufacturers. Two of the most popular manufacturers are Mountain House and AlpineAire. As with any food manufacturer, their products differ in terms of taste, energy distribution, protein, and sodium content. Many of the items from both companies have been tested under field conditions for up to 30 days, and the acceptability varies from person to person. What is important is that a ration that will providing adequate energy and CHO is chosen.

Future Rations

Current and future initiatives will continue to explore technologies for continual improvement of all military rations. The end result will be a highly acceptable product that provides the Warfighter with sustained energy, mental alertness, and eat-on-the-move capability. The Department of Defense Combat Feeding Program strives to uncover new solutions and capabilities that support U.S. military objectives.

14 Eating Globally

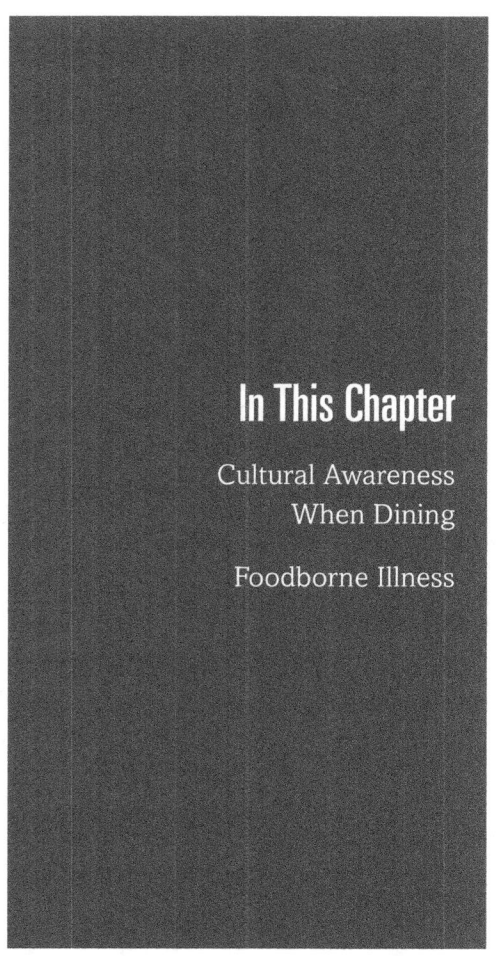

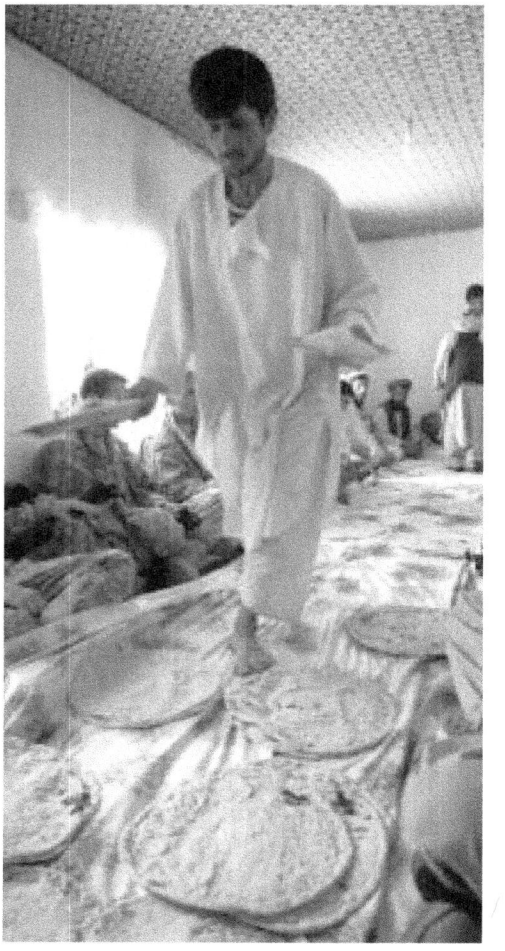

Key Points

- Be aware of cultural differences including types of food and proper eating utensils.

- Avoid foodborne illnesses by taking extra precautions: stay away from typical foods associated with foodborne illnesses.

- Make wise food and beverage selections when eating on the economy.

- Drinking contaminated water may severely affect your health: purify your water!

- Carry Pepto-Bismol and seek medical treatment for symptoms from contaminated foods or beverages.

Most operations take place on the soil of other countries and each country, region and even town may have their own culture. Foods are a large part of any culture and sharing meals can be a great way to interact and form relationships with the locals. Enjoying the local chef's food is important, but some cultural foods or approaches to preparing meals can lead to illness for those unaccustomed to local practices. This chapter will discuss cultural differences, foods that are and are not eaten based on religious beliefs, and how to avoid foodborne illnesses.

Cultural Awareness When Dining

Cultural awareness means recognizing, understanding, appreciating and respecting the different perspectives and customs of one's own culture and the culture of others. Culture involves language, beliefs, religion, values, behaviors, food preferences, and eating habits, and more.

Always be aware of the host country's surroundings and become familiar with the local customs and cultures to avoid stereotypes, prejudice, and insulting the host, particularly when it comes to dining.

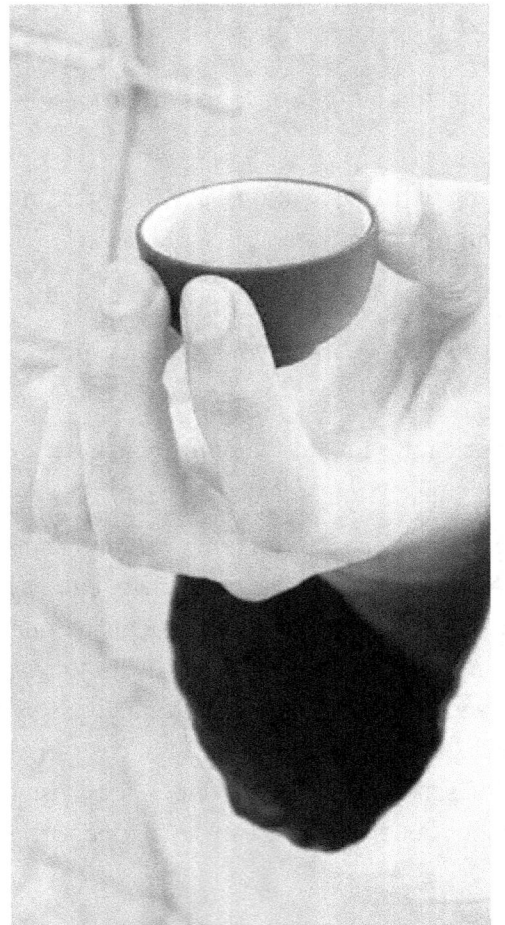

As you deploy to different regions of the world, learn the eating customs and enjoy the dining experiences.

Cultural differences in eating habits may be as simple as using a fork and knife in Europe and the U.S. versus chopsticks in Asia or fingers in other countries. In some parts of the world a common plate is shared versus individual plates in other countries. In some countries, the right hand is considered the clean hand and is used for eating.

Some cultures eat primarily vegetarian meals and in other countries almost anything that moves is considered edible. Don't be surprised if you are fed lamb, goat, horse, dog, camel, or monkey. In many cultures all parts of the animal are consumed or used in cooking (brains, organs, feet, intestines, etc).

Different foods are used throughout the world in holiday and ceremonial meals. A few additional customs related to eating are listed; however, prior to deployment and throughout deployments, the local eating customs should be learned and respected.

Know the Local Customs

Don't be surprised when visiting another country to find many customs that we as Americans have never heard of. Do your homework before being deployed.

Think Before You Act....

The Basics

- Know whether punctuality is or is not emphasized.

- Use the appropriate customary greeting (hand shake, bow, etc).

- Learn if it is customary to bring a hostess gift, food, or beverages to the social gathering. In some cultures it is very impolite and implies that you are paying for the meal.

- Don't criticize.

- Know whether it is customary to clean your plate or leave a little food. In some cultures, cleaning your plate indicates hunger and poverty.

- Eating may be as much for social interactions as it is for nourishment. Do not rush through your meals.

- Do not be wasteful or gorge yourself. Your host may have gone to great expense to prepare an extravagant meal. Remember that it probably has been quite costly, and what you consume may cost a week's salary or feed his/her family for an extended period of time.

Who Eats First?

- Be aware of who should begin the meal—is it the host, the guest or the person of highest status?

Appetizers

- Some countries serve a salad with a meal, while others serve it as an appetizer or following the main meal.

Soup

- Hot soups may be eaten after every dinner meal.
- Some foods are very spicy. The small green bean in the soup may actually be a hot pepper.
- Is slurping soup considered rude or acceptable and a sign of enjoyment?

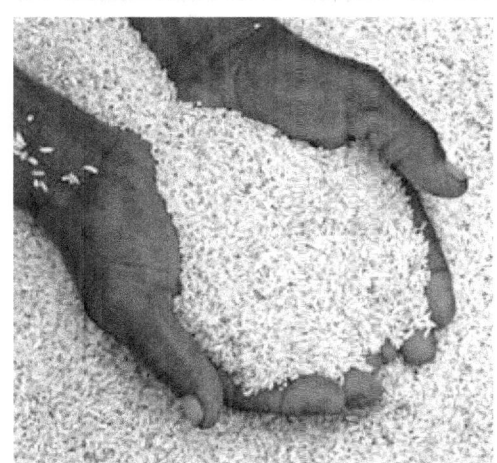

Meats/Fish

- Pork is not eaten by Muslims for religious reasons.
- Christians keep dogs, cats, and horses for pets, while others may eat them for dinner.
- Fish is typically a neutral food.

Not Just Any Rice

- In Thailand, it is believed that rice has a sacred essence, and it is important to avoid inappropriate usage or disposal of rice.

Dessert

- Desserts may or may not be a typical part of the meal.

Beverages

- Coffee and tea may be served with sugar and cream already added; it may be very sweet.

Food Offerings

- Foods are typically offered when visiting and it may be rude to turn down a beverage.
- If you are the host in a developing country, serve something when others

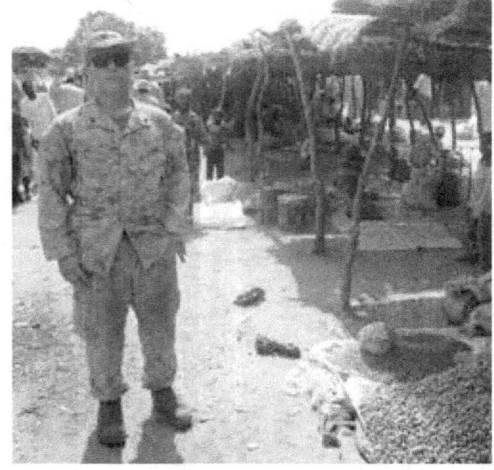

visit your office or, as you would be treated when visiting their office.

- Try not to refuse beverages and food when offered.

What Time is Dinner Being Served?

- Meals are eaten at different hours of the day.

Eating Instruments

- Some countries use the fork as the primary eating utensil and others use the spoon, hand or chopsticks.

- Be familiar with the use of chopsticks and whether they are used for the entire meal or only with the appetizers.

- Follow the host's lead. Is rice pushed from the rice bowl directly into the mouth or eaten with a utensil?

- Is soup consumed with a spoon or drunk directly from the bowl?

- Bosnian Muslims, unlike Arab Muslims, use their left hand when eating or passing objects. In Saudi, the left hand is considered the dirty, toilet hand.

Proper Dress Attire

- Dress appropriately and not too informally.

- In certain cultures, it is important to remove shoes at the door.

Paying the bill

- Paying for a meal is generally done by the one inviting.

- Paying is considered an honor.

Good Ideas

- Become aware of local food taboos.

- Avoid yawning at the table.

- Excessive or loud talking and joking during a meal may be considered rude.

- Don't criticize.

- It may be impolite to stare at someone while they are eating.

- Become familiar with local foods that have traditional medicinal qualities or are used as folk medicine.

Foodborne Illness

Situations may arise where food choices are extremely limited, like when deploying to austere environments in developing countries. In addition, when an international host presents foods and beverages, it may be difficult to refuse what is offered.

It is very important to be courteous of local customs and culture surrounding food preparation and consumption.

When placed in situations where food and beverage choices are limited, a few basic principles should be followed to avoid foodborne illness. To maintain operational readiness and prevent the common gastrointestinal distress or "traveler's diarrhea," paying close attention to what you eat and drink is essential.

Foodborne illnesses are "infections" caused by consuming food or water that contains selected bacteria, viruses, parasites, and/or various harmful toxins, such as pesticides, poisonous mushrooms, and arsenic. The risk of infection varies depending on where the food is eaten—from fairly low in private homes to high in food purchased from street vendors.

The more than 250 different foodborne diseases have many different symptoms, so there is no one "syndrome" that describes foodborne illness. However, the "culprit" enters the body through the gastrointestinal tract, where the first symptoms—nausea, vomiting, abdominal cramps, and diarrhea—appear.

Foods Associated with Foodborne Illness

Certain foods are typically associated with foodborne illnesses. Raw foods, particularly of animal origin, are a major concern if served. Stay clear of:

- Raw meat and poultry.

- Ground beef and raw eggs.

- Unpasteurized milk or fresh squeezed fruit juice.

- Raw shellfish, including oysters.

- Raw fruits and vegetables.

- Salads.

- Alfalfa and bean sprouts.

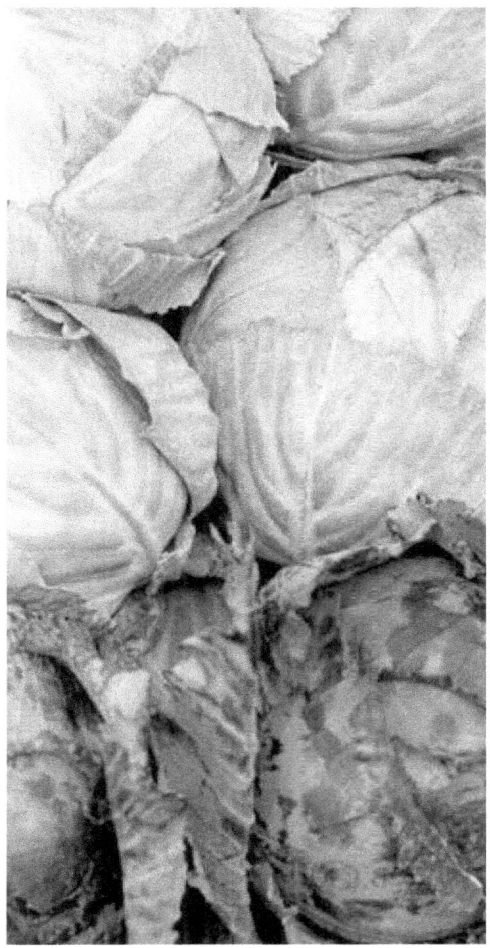

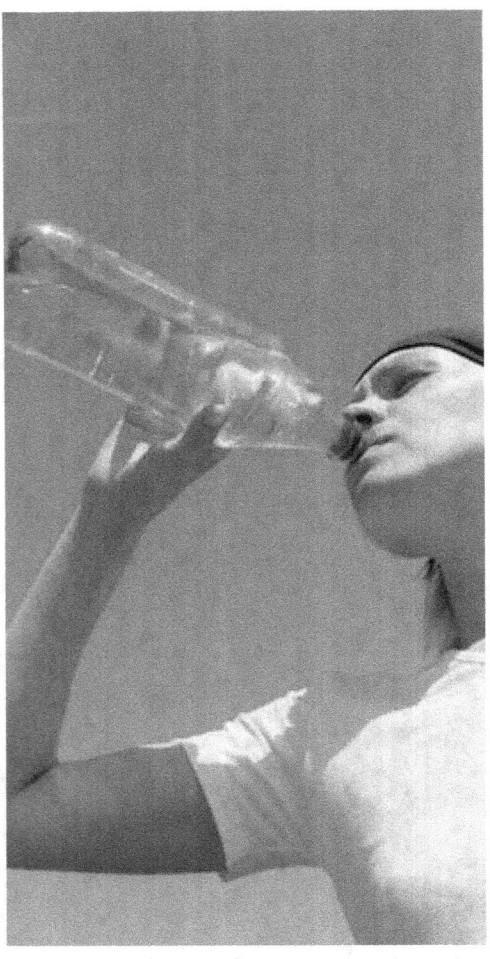

Drink only bottled water from approved sources.

Fruits and vegetables can be just as poisonous as raw meat and fish. Washing can decrease, but not eliminate, contamination, in part because the water may be contaminated, so consumers can do little to protect themselves.

Making Wise Food Selections

It is possible to make wise food selections; eating with caution may save a few days of discomfort. Remember these basic tips:

- Food that has been cooked and is still hot is usually safe.

- Some fish is not guaranteed to be safe, even when cooked, because of the presence of toxins.

- When eating at street vendors ensure foods are cooked in front of you. Do not select those that may have been cooked hours ago.

- Avoid raw ingredients, such as fresh vegetables. Fresh salads, even in many restaurants, can be contaminated due to the use of human waste for fertilizer.

- If offered a beverage, choose a safe one, such as boiled water, hot beverages (such as coffee or tea) made with boiled water, canned or bottled carbonated beverages, beer, and wine.

- Avoid ice in beverages. Ice may be made from contaminated water.

- Use purified or bottled water to brush your teeth. Do not even use small amounts of untreated water for rinsing your mouth.

- Fresh fruit and vegetables with skins are usually fine if cleaned thoroughly. Scrub the skin with purified water or soap and water and then peel. If not cleaned, the contamination may be transferred to the fruit or vegetable during the peeling process.

- Avoid fruits and vegetables that have already been peeled.

- Most bakery products are safe, but avoid those with a cream or meat filling.

- Order hamburgers cooked well-done and without lettuce and tomato.

- Avoid milk and juice that has not been pasteurized.

- Foods that have been deep fried or cooked thoroughly are acceptable to eat.

- Staple items such as pasta, rice, potatoes or other root vegetables that have been boiled or cooked over high heat, are safe items.

- Do not consume foods left at room temperature for over 4 hours.

- When eating eggs, ensure that the yolk is cooked until firm.

- High salt, high sugar, and high acid levels keep bacteria from growing, which is why salted meats, jam, and pickled vegetables are traditional preserved foods.

Water Purification

"Montezuma's Revenge" from contaminated drinking water can occur anywhere. Chemical disinfection can be achieved with either iodine or chlorine. These chemicals may not make water taste like bottled water from home, but it will decrease the risks of drinking untreated water.

The disinfection capabilities of iodine have been recognized for many years and iodine tablets are widely used as an emergency drinking water disinfectant.

- Add two iodine tablets to a 1.1 quart (1 liter) of water, wait 5 minutes, shake, loosen the cap, and then wait 30 more minutes before drinking.

Chlorine is also a reliable water disinfectant. Water purification tablets issued by the military that contain chlorine kill giardia lamblia cysts, bacteria, viruses, and other harmful micro-organisms, and remove sediment.

- Add 1 water disinfectant tablet (600 mg/1.4% available chlorine) to 1.10 qt (1 L) of water at temperatures of 77°F (25°C). Add two tablets (2.8% available chlorine) at 41°F (5°C) for the same purpose.

Lastly, boiling is a most reliable method to make water safe to drink.

- Bring water to a vigorous boil, and then allow it to cool.

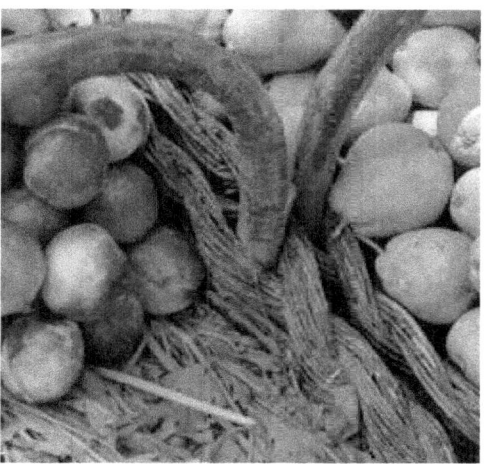

Water purification tablets are intended for clarifying and disinfecting polluted/suspended water to make it safe for drinking.

Preventive and Treatment Measures for Foodborne Illness

Many different foodborne diseases may be prevented or treated. One preventive approach is Pepto-Bismol. Pepto-Bismol can be taken before and during international travel to help prevent diarrhea. The usual approach is to take two ounces of the pink medication four times daily, or two tablets, four times daily, for no longer than three weeks.

Side effects of Pepto-Bismol may include temporary blackening of tongue and stools, occasional nausea and constipation, and rarely, ringing in the ears. Do not take Pepto-Bismol if you have an aspirin allergy, renal insufficiency, gout, or are taking anticoagulants, probenecid (Benemid, Probalan), or methotrexate (Rheumatrex).

The treatment of foodborne illnesses depends on the symptoms. Illnesses that cause primarily diarrhea or vomiting can lead to dehydration more body fluids and salts (electrolytes) are lost than taken in.

The treatment of traveler's diarrhea requires the replacement of lost fluids and salts. This is best achieved by use of an oral rehydration solution, such as the World Health Organization's oral rehydration salts (ORS) solution. Another solution to electrolyte losses may be the new SportStrips, which deliver electrolytes directly through cells in the mouth. These SportStrips, by Health Sports, have not been tested, but do provide essential electrolytes independent of the gastrointestinal tract and may be helpful for gastrointestinal distress.

ORS packets, available at stores or pharmacies in almost all developing countries, are similar to Pedialyte. ORS is prepared by adding one packet to boiled or treated water. Packet instructions should be followed carefully to ensure that the salts are added to the correct volume of water. Sports drinks, such as Gatorade, do not replace the losses correctly and should not be used for the treatment of diarrheal illness. Electrolyte sport strips (http://www.enlytenstrips.com) should allow for rapid absorption of electrolytes and would be tastier than ORS.

For those who don't listen to warnings, Pepto-Bismol and other preparations of bismuth subsalicylate can reduce the duration and severity of simple diarrhea. Pepto-Bismol decreases diarrhea frequency and shortens the duration of the illness. An over-the-counter antidiarrheal medication, such as Lomotil or Imodium, can decrease the number of diarrheal stools, but can cause complications in people with serious infections. An antidiarrheal medication may provide symptomatic relief, but these medications should not be used with a high fever or bloody stools because they may make the illness worse.

Antibiotics (which require a prescription) may shorten the length of illness. The CDC does not recommend the use of antibiotics to prevent traveler's diarrhea because they can sometimes cause additional problems. Consult a doctor before taking these medications.

When to Consult a Health Care Provider

Foodborne illnesses can be dangerous and must be treated seriously. Consult a health care provider when diarrheal illness is accompanied by:

- High fever (temperature over 101.5°F, measured orally).
- Blood in the stools.
- Prolonged vomiting that prevents keeping liquids down.
- Signs of dehydration, including a decrease in urination, dry mouth and throat, and feeling dizzy upon standing.
- Diarrhea that lasts more than 3 days.

Do not be surprised if antibiotics are not prescribed for diarrheal illness. Diarrheal illness caused by viruses will improve in two or three days without antibiotic therapy. Other treatments can alleviate the symptoms, and hand washing can prevent others from becoming sick.

Whenever possible, you should consult a health care professional for foodborne illness.

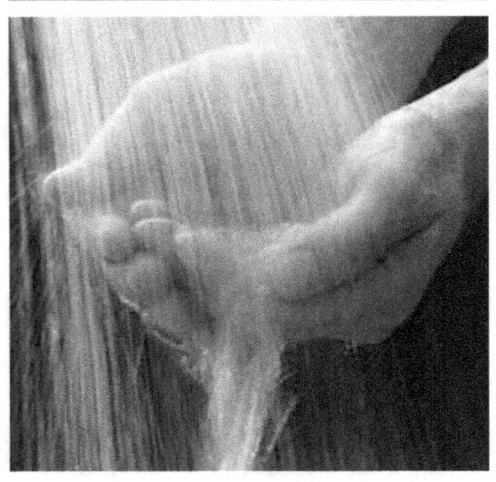

Careful hand washing can curtail and potentially prevent the spread of infection to other people.

15 Mission Nutrition for Combat Effectiveness

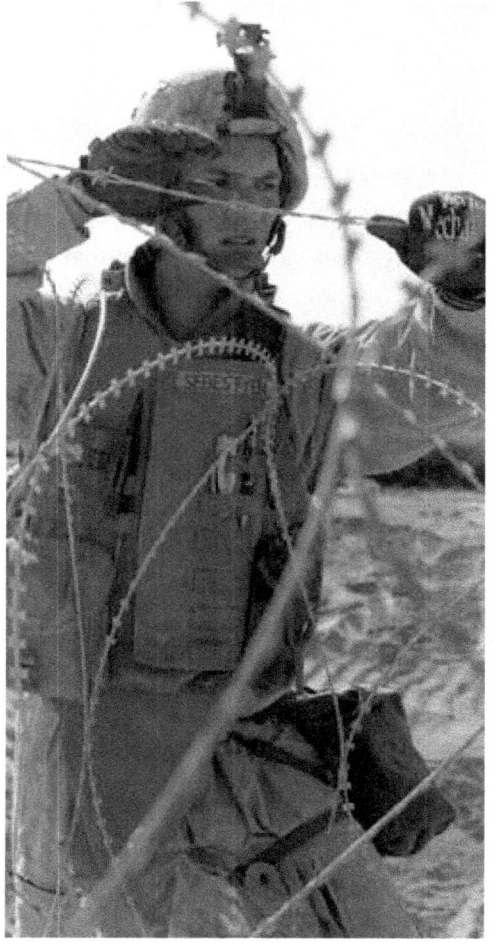

Key Points

- Inadequate energy intake and/or dehydration can result in fatigue and impaired performance during combat.

- Improper eating and sleeping due to all night and high op-tempo missions can be detrimental to overall health.

- Eating before night operations should be planned accordingly to prevent fatigue.

- Various environmental exposures (i.e. heat, cold, and altitude) can alter combat effectiveness if nutritional needs and hydration are not met appropriately.

- Energy and fluid requirements are typically higher than normal during combat and combat-simulated scenarios.

The synergistic relationship between adequate fueling and operational performance on the battlefield cannot be underestimated when it comes to mission success. Operators of equipment like humvees, helicopters, and submarines require high performance fuels to operate effectively. In some instances fueling options are limited, but meeting energy and fluid requirements whenever possible is critical. This chapter describes various fueling options when exposed to various environmental and logistical extremes. As Napoleon Bonaparte stated, "An army marches on its stomach."

Nutritional Readiness Before Missions

Warfighters must be prepared for deployments at any time. Immediately before such events, they may find themselves in the field or under lock down on base. Regardless, the two main nutritional considerations for readiness before missions are:

- Maximizing glycogen stores.

- Being well-hydrated.

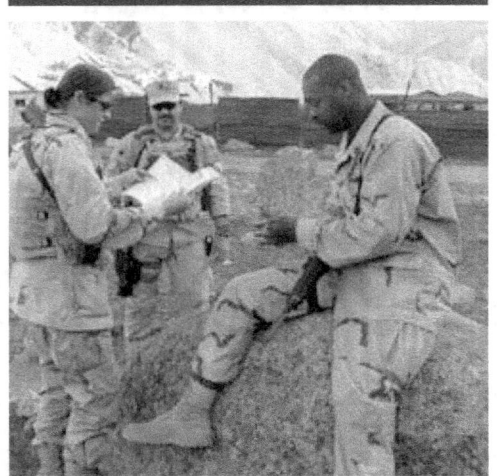

Several Days Before a Mission

The average, lean, 175-pound man has approximately 1,800 calories of CHO stored as glycogen in liver and muscle, and 75,000 to 150,000 calories stored as fat or adipose tissue. Despite these large energy stores of fat, CHO is still the preferred fuels, and glycogen depletion will compromise physical and mental performance. Low glycogen stores = fatigue. A diet rich in CHO for several days before a mission will increase liver and muscle glycogen stores, and thereby ensure adequate fuels stores.

Timing and Composition of Pre-Mission Meals

The purpose of the pre-mission meal is to ensure adequate glycogen stores and maintain blood sugar. Every Warfighter should know his own tolerance for timing of meals and what patterns are needed to sustain performance. In general, intense physical activities demand a longer time period after meal ingestion to allow for digestion and minimize gastrointestinal distress.

Eat 2–4 grams of CHO per pound body weight, but no more than 400 grams, 3–4 hours before a sustained operation.

A pre-mission meal should provide a minimum of fat, since it takes longer to digest than CHO. CHO beverages and CHO/protein drinks are excellent choices if taken four hours before the start of a mission. Liquids are digested and absorbed more rapidly than solids, but personal choice is important. Avoid a high protein meal because it is harder to digest than CHO, and is not a readily available source of energy.

Sustained Night Operations

Night exercises require acute cognitive awareness and the ability to react quickly to sudden and potential compromised situations. Sustained Operations (SUSOPS) are work periods of 24 hours or more that usually result in physical and mental fatigue as well as sleep loss. In contrast, Continuous Operations (CONOPS) are periods of uninterrupted activity of "normal shift length" followed by sufficient sleep. Missions include both SUSOPS and CONOPS, which can frequently result in fatigue and sleep deprivation. Nutritional interventions can partially offset the detrimental effects of fatigue and sleep deprivation on physical and mental performance. The nutritional interventions most effective include:

- Carbohydrate intake
- Hydration status
- Caffeine intake

CHO Intake

As noted earlier, a high CHO diet is needed to maintain muscle glycogen stores and blood glucose. A diet that provides 50 to 70% of energy from CHO, 10 to 20% from protein and 20 to 35% of calories from fat is important for SUSOPS. High CHO snacks and/or CHO-containing fluid replacement beverages providing 15–30 g of CHO/hour will also help to maintain blood glucose and delay fatigue during strenuous prolonged missions. When blood glucose levels fall, hypoglycemia results causing performance to drop rapidly, and you will be incapable to continue the workload you initially started at.

Table 15–1. Symptoms of Hypoglycemia	
Headache	Weakness
Dizziness	Fatigue
Blurred vision	Sweating
Confusion	Unconsciousness

Portable foods that are easily accessible should always be included in a Warfighter "kit." Quick eating foods that can fit conveniently in uniform pockets were presented in Chapter 8, Healthy Snacking. Additional foods include vacuum packed tuna or chicken with crackers and pocket sandwiches. Avoid foods that are high in the amino acid, tryptophan, since tryptophan promotes sleep.

Table 15–2. Foods High in Tryptophan	
Dairy products and Eggs	Soy products
Seafood	Whole grains
Poultry	Rice
Meats	Hazelnuts, Peanuts
Beans and Lentils	Sesame seeds, sunflower seeds

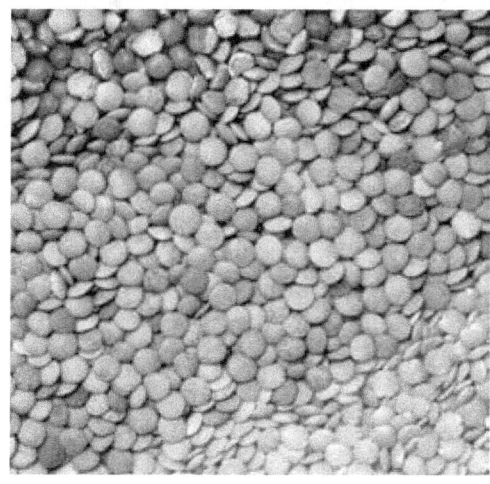

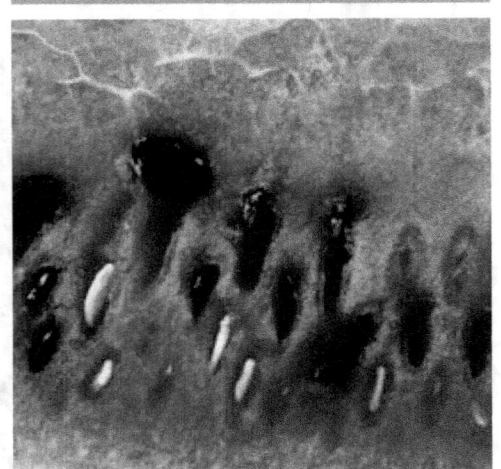

Hydration Status

Since water is critical for maintaining optimal operational performance as well as maintaining good general health, proper daily water intake is one of the most important factors for Warfighters. In 2004, the Institute of Medicine updated the adequate intake (AI) for water to 3.7 liters, or nearly one gallon of water, per day for men over the age of 19. Individuals typically need 1 milliliter of water for every kcal consumed. Warfighters usually have fluid needs greater than the recommended guidelines because of intense training, working in high humidity, extreme temperatures, and austere environments.

When possible, select fluids that contribute not only fluids, but also vitamins and minerals.

Fluid balance can be maintained with beverages containing water, such as juice, milk, coffee, tea, soda, and foods. Fruits and vegetables contain an upwards of 70%–90% water, whereas meats, dairy products and grain products consist of 30%–50%.

Beverages consumed in the heat should be no more than 8% CHO—or less than 19 grams/8 oz.

The need for electrolyte replacement in the field may be very great under warm and hot weather conditions, and during military exercises involving high mobility and strenuous physical work lasting 60 minutes or longer. When water is the only fluid available, the electrolyte SportStrips, a new product on the market, may be very useful. The SportStrips, which provide sodium and potassium, are inserted into the mouth between the gums and cheek and should be absorbed very quickly. The gastrointestinal tract is not required for absorption and as such, may be important for other conditions, such as dehydration from diarrhea. The effectiveness of this product is under review, but appears promising for military applications because of its simplicity and ease of transporting.

Dehydration can result in a loss of appetite.

Fluid replacement beverages with CHO are suggested during extended missions; however, the amount of CHO should be lower than usual so that the fluid/water is rapidly absorbed.

Caffeine Intake

It is well-recognized that caffeine increases alertness and may delay fatigue during extended operations. However, the effective dose may vary, depending on habitual caffeine intake and sensitivity to caffeine. Caffeine is less effective for those who routinely consume large amounts. For caffeine to be effective, it should be consumed on an irregular basis.

A common dose shown to be effective for maintaining performance and vigilance is 200 mg. Although less may also be effective, the military has prepared "Stay Alert" gum, which contains 100 mg per chicklet. The current recommendation is to take 200 mg every two hours, for up to eight hours straight to help with alertness during operations. A regular dosing is needed because the effects of caffeine typically wear off within six hours.

Caffeine-rich beverages and foods are among the most popular forms of nutrition to help Warfighters maintain alertness at night. However, most products containing caffeine do not list amounts of caffeine on Nutrition Facts Labels. Manufacturers are not required to list caffeine amounts on labels, so the consumer can only determine the caffeine content by recognizing caffeine effects.

Weight loss in the field is common, but may impair mental and physical performance.

Nutritional Readiness During Missions

Four major nutrition-related issues encountered in the field are:

- Inadequate ration consumption.
- Inadequate energy intake.
- Dehydration.
- Gastrointestinal complaints.

Rations

One of the biggest problems with eating rations is that it gets boring! Monotony and lack of time to eat contribute to decreased ration intake and weight loss. Therefore, it is important to consume as much of the field ration as possible to maintain performance and health.

Eat part of each ration item to obtain all the essential nutrients.

Limit use of non-issue food items as meal/ration substitutes since they may be lacking in several important nutrients. Use these items as snacks to supplement daily rations. Also pack high CHO items, such as crackers, dried fruits, trail mixes, sports bars, and like (see Chapter 8 for snack ideas). Experiment beforehand to see what suits you best. When planning to use high CHO bars, check the fat content, because if the fat content is greater than 3 g/100 calories it may slow down absorption and can cause cramps.

The new First Strike Ration, which provides an average of 2,900 kcal per day, is great for missions, except that additional CHO must be provided to meet CHO needs. Table 3 provides the content of the three menus. This new ration takes up less space and weighs approximately 50% less than three MREs.

Table 15–3. Menus for First Strike Ration		
Menu 1	**Menu 2**	**Menu 3**
Filled French toast pocket	Brown sugar cinnamon toaster pastry	Lemon poppyseed pound cake
Bacon cheddar pocket sandwich	Italian pocket sandwich	Honey BBQ beef pocket sandwich
Pepperoni pocket sandwich	Chunk chicken	Albacore tuna
Jalapeno cheese spread	Tortillas	Tortillas
Wheat snack bread	Peanut butter	Cheese spread, plain
ERGO drink	Cracker, plain	Cracker, plain
ERGO drink	ERGO drink	ERGO drink
First Strike!™ mocha	ERGO drink	ERGO drink
First Strike!™ chocolate	First Strike!™ apple cinnamon	First Strike!™ mocha
Peanut butter dessert bar	First Strike!™ cranraspberry	First Strike!™ cranraspberry
Beef snack, sweet BBQ	Dessert bar, mocha	Dessert bar, chocolate banana nut
Beef snack, teriyaki	Beef snack, sweet BBQ	Beef snack, sweet BBQ

Table 15–3. Menus for First Strike Ration		
Menu 1	**Menu 2**	**Menu 3**
CHO enhanced applesauce	Beef snack, teriyaki	Beef snack, teriyaki
Nut fruit mix	CHO enhanced applesauce	CHO enhanced applesauce
Caffeinated gum	Nut fruit mix	Nut fruit mix
	Caffeinated gum	Caffeinated gum
	Mayonnaise, fat-free	Mayonnaise, fat-free
	Hot sauce	Hot sauce
Access C	**Access B**	**Access A**
Apple cider	Lemon tea	Coffee
Towelette	Towelette	Cream substitute
Salt	Salt	Sugar
Matches	Matches	Towelette
Tissue	Tissue	Salt

Each menu comes with a zip-lock pouch, 2 towelettes, and a spoon.

If possible, drink 25 to 60 grams of CHO/hour to maintain blood glucose.

Dehydration

Dehydration occurs when sweat and urine losses are not replaced by drinking water and other fluid replacement products. It can occur at altitude, in the cold, in the heat, during diving, and even under conditions of low physical activity. Mild dehydration can decrease appetite and cause lethargy. It should be avoided at all costs

Water and other fluids should be consumed when thirsty. At least 4 L should be consumed each day—more when the environment is hot.

Gastrointestinal Complaints

Changes in diet, dehydration, too much fiber, poor sanitary conditions, contaminated food, unfamiliar bacteria, and/or stress may result in diarrhea or constipation in the field. Ensure adequate hydration at all times,

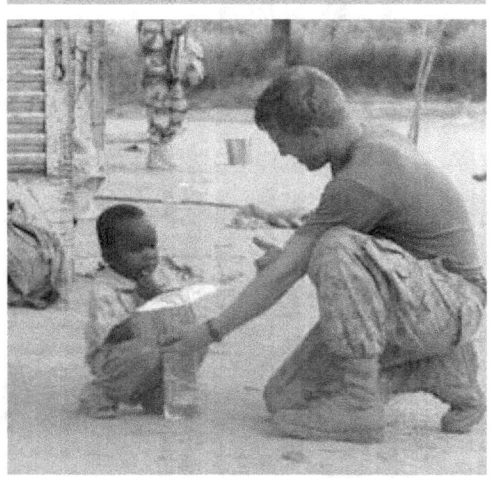

and avoid new non-issue foods whenever possible. Chapter 14, Eating Locally discusses approaches to mitigating gastrointestinal distress.

Missions in the Heat

Repetitive movement along difficult terrain with heavy gear, such as during land warfare operations, is strenuous under any environmental condition, but particularly arduous with extreme heat and humidity. Land warfare scenarios where Warfighters carry heavy loads or injured comrades increase overall effort and energy expenditure, as well as fluid and electrolyte needs. The major concerns during operations in a warm/ hot environment are fluid and electrolyte balance. Working or exercising in the heat exacerbates water and electrolyte loss through sweating. The amount of sweat and fluid lost depends on:

- Environmental temperature and humidity.

- Work rate.

- Fitness level and acclimatization.

- Volume and rate of fluid replacement.

When the same task carried out in thermoneutral environment is performed in a hot environment, energy requirements are slightly increased due to the increased work of maintaining thermal balance. When living/ working in temperatures ranging from 86 to 104° F (30 to 40° C), energy intakes typically increase by 10%, unless activity level decreases accordingly.

If 4,000 kcal/day are required, a 10% increase in energy would = 4,000 x 0.10 or +400 kcal/day.

Goal: Consume 4,400 kcal/day.

Tip: If activity levels decrease, no extra energy is needed!

High work rates in hot, humid surroundings can significantly increase fluid and electrolyte losses. Losses of one to two quarts per hour or even more are likely when special clothing, such as chemical protective gear, and/or body armor is worn. The highest sweat rates reported are over five quarts per hour. That is a lot of fluid.

Fluids—Drink Early and Drink Often

Starting any operation without being adequately hydrated may increase the risk of performance mishaps. Some believe that relying on thirst is adequate for sustaining hydration, whereas others believe that thirst itself is an indicator of dehydration. For certain, failure to replace lost fluids from sweating will result in dehydration and possibly heat injury. Always drink when thirsty.

Although forced drinking is recommended throughout training in a warm environment to ensure adequate fluid replacement and performance, this is not always wise. Too much water can result in hyponatremia. A pre-determined drinking schedule is recommended to ensure enough fluids are being consumed: some type of beverage should be consumed with all meals and snacks.

Drink 1–2 cups of fluid every 30 minutes.

Drinking more than 4 cups per 60 minutes may be *too much* to absorb!

In the field when it is difficult, if not impossible, to obtain a body weight, urine color should be used to gauge hydration status.

One pound of weight lost requires 2.25 cups or 0.5 quarts of fluid to restore fluid balance.

A fluid loss of 2% body weight can impair physical performance and mood, decrease appetite, and increase the risk of heat injuries. A 5% loss of body weight can decrease work performance by 30%. This amount of water loss is a serious threat to overall health.

Monitoring Hydration in the Field

Monitor hydration status by inspecting urine color.

Dark yellow or smelly urine suggests some degree of dehydration; fluid consumption should be increased until urine becomes pale yellow. If taking B vitamins, urine may be bright yellow, not pale, regardless of hydration status.

Example:

A WF weighs 175 pounds.

A 4% weight loss would be 175 x 0.04 = 7.0 lbs.

Goal: Stay above 168 lbs.

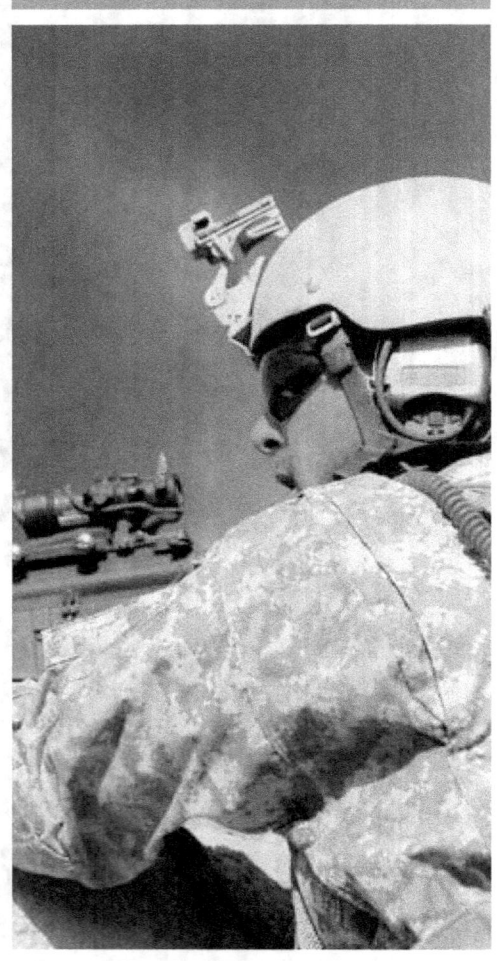

Electrolyte Balance

Excessive loss of electrolytes (i.e., sodium, potassium) from sweating can lead to muscle cramping or severe medical problems. Being in excellent physical condition will help minimize electrolyte losses, but athletes given free access to water when exercising in the heat replace only one half to two thirds of their fluid losses. Also, camelbacks are routinely used to stay hydrated, but since they provide water alone, electrolyte balance may be compromised. To maintain electrolyte snacks that contain sodium and potassium, fluids with electrolytes, electrolyte SportStrips or electrolytes in the form of gels and blocks may be needed during and after missions. Electrolytes should offset hyponatremia.

Fluids alone may not be adequate for restoring or maintaining electrolyte balance, because there is an upper limit to how much sodium and potassium should be provided in a beverage.

Table 15-4. Upper Limits for Sodium and Potassium in Fluid Replacement Beverages During Heat Stress		
Units	Sodium	Potassium
mg/8 oz	165	46
mg/L	690	195
mEq/8 oz	7.2	1.2

Check labels to ensure that beverages provide no more than indicated in the chart above. The National Academy of Sciences recommends that chloride be the only "anion" (negatively charged electrolyte) accompanying sodium and potassium, and no other electrolytes are recommended. Typically, magnesium and calcium are included, but the amounts are well below recommended upper limits.

In addition, foods that naturally provide sodium and potassium should be selected. Dried fruits are optimal food choices for potassium. For example, a small box of raisins provides 322 mg of potassium. Even if heat acclimatization has occurred, it is important to understand the importance of salt: 200–400 milligrams of sodium can be lost per pound of sweat, along with sodium excreted in urine. Adding salt to foods (1/2 teaspoon provides 1,200 milligrams) or including sodium-rich foods in the diet will help retain water and avoid a sodium deficit. Sodium is the most critical electrolyte for maintaining fluid balance.

Table 15-5. Sodium Content of Foods

Food	Serving Size	Sodium (mg)
Bacon	3 oz	621
Canned chicken soup	1 cup	850
Cheese, American	1 oz	304
Cornflakes	1 cup	298
Cottage cheese	½ cup	459
Deli ham	1 oz	341
Deli turkey breast	1 oz	335
Olives, black	5 large	192
Peanut butter smooth, salted	2 Tbsp	147
Peanuts, dry roasted, salted	3 oz	691
Pickles, dill	1 large	1,731
Potato chips	1 oz	183
Pretzels	1 oz	486
Sardines	3 oz	429
Sauerkraut	½ cup	780
Soy sauce	1 tsp	304
Table salt	1 tsp	2,358
Tortilla chips	3 oz	669

Table 15-6. Potassium Content of Foods

Food	Serving Size	Potassium (mg)
Apricots, dried	10 halves	407
Avocados, raw	1 oz	180
Bananas, raw	1 cup	594

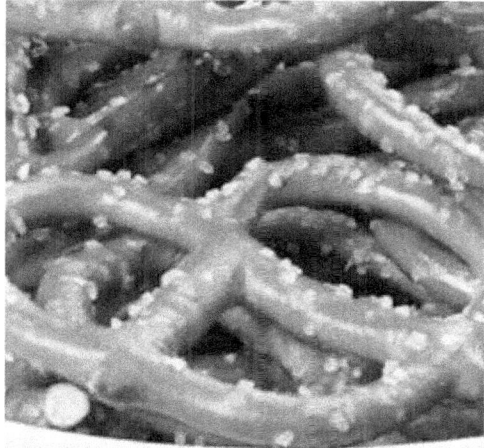

Table 15-6. Potassium Content of Foods		
Food	**Serving Size**	**Potassium (mg)**
Cantaloupe	1 cup	494
Dates, dry	5 dates	271
Figs, dry	2 figs	271
Kiwi fruit, raw	1 medium	252
Lima beans	1 cup	955
Melons, honeydew	1 cup	461
Milk, fat-free or skim	1 cup	407
Nectarines	1 medium	288
Orange juice	1 cup	496
Oranges	1 orange	237
Pears, fresh	1 pear	208
Peanuts, dry roasted, without salt	1 ounce	187
Potato, baked, with skin	1 potato	1,081
Prune juice	1 cup	707
Prunes, dried	1 cup	828
Raisins	1 cup	1,089
Spinach, cooked	1 cup	839
Tomato sauce	1 cup	909
Winter squash	1 cup	896
Yogurt, plain, skim milk	8 oz	579

Missions in the Cold

Exposure to a cold environment seriously challenges the human body. Blood vessels tighten to conserve heat and shivering is initiated to generate heat and guard against hypothermia (a dangerously low core body temperature). Side effects of these responses are: an increase in urine output and an increase in energy metabolism. Therefore, the most important nutritional considerations for a cold environment are:

- Energy intake.

- Glycogen stores.

- Fluid status.

- Vitamin and mineral needs.

Energy Intake

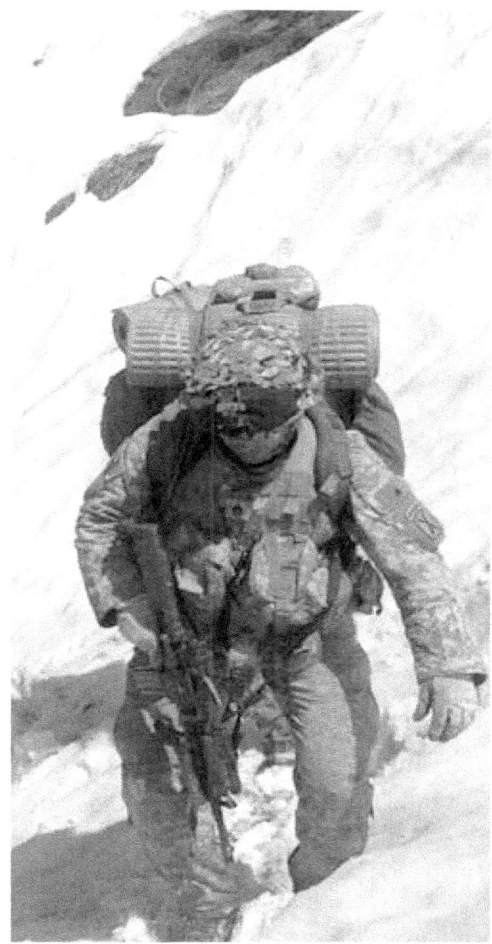

Energy requirements can increase 25–50% during cold weather operations as compared to warm weather operations.

Cold weather increases energy requirements significantly. Factors that increase caloric intake include:

- Added exertion due to wearing heavy gear.

- Shivering, which can increase resting metabolic rate by two to four times the normal level.

- Increased activity associated with traveling over snow and icy terrain.

- Increased activity to keep warm.

Many studies have shown that Warfighters tend to progressively lose weight when conducting two to three week field exercises in the cold. Because significant weight loss can result in fatigue and performance decrements, energy intake should meet the increased energy demands.

Energy expenditure for Warfighters during periods of physical exertion in the cold may range between 4,200 and 5,000 kcal/day. Although CHO is critical, a diet that provides 35% of the energy as fat may be necessary to match energy needs. It is important to remember that both fat and CHO are important energy sources in a cold environment.

Ideally, during cold weather operations, 50–60% of energy should come from CHO, 30–35% from fat, and 10–20% from protein: high CHO snacks should be eaten between meals. A high protein diet is not advised as it may increase fluid requirements.

Missions in cold weather require foods that produce heat. Foods high in CHO produce more heat through digestion than either fat or protein. Hot beverages, such as cocoa, provide CHO and other warm beverages, to in-

Example:

WF require ~4,000 kcal/day

A 25% increase in energy would
= 4,000 x 0.25 or +1,000 kcal

Goal: Consume 5,000 kcal/day

clude coffee, teas and broth, increase body temperature, enhance mental awareness and provide comfort.

Eat high CHO snacks frequently.

Glycogen Stores

Prior to deploying to a cold environment, the pre-mission diet should ensure that glycogen stores are optimized. Likewise, a high CHO diet is preferred during cold exposure, as CHO are needed to replenish glycogen being used to maintain core temperature. Thus, regular meals and snacks providing CHO should be eaten to maintain CHO intake. Including a liquid or solid CHO supplement may be critical for maintaining energy balance and performance.

A minimum of 400 grams of CHO is necessary in the cold.

Fluid Status

Becoming dehydrated in cold environments is easy because of the cold-induced increase in urine output, increased fluid losses through breathing, involuntary reduction in fluid intake, and sweating. Because dehydration decreases performance and potentially may lead to various medical problems, maintaining fluid status by drinking plenty of fluids and monitoring hydration is absolutely critical.

Table 15-7. Tips for Maintaining Fluid Status
Force yourself to drink 2–4 cups of warm fluid at hourly intervals.
Avoid alcoholic beverages: alcohol tends to increase heat and urine losses.
Drink beverages with CHO to increase energy intake.
Don't eat snow without first melting and purifying it.
Moderate caffeine consumption.

Beverages containing 5–8% CHO
and some electrolytes are best.
Drinking 1 to 2 cups per 30
minutes is recommended.

Vitamin and Mineral Needs

The requirements for some vitamins and minerals increase when working in the cold due to increases in energy metabolism (example: thiamin) or urinary losses (example: magnesium, zinc). The amount by which daily vitamin and mineral needs may increase above the DRI during cold weather operations are shown in Table 8. These amounts are based on intake data from field studies, urinary excretion of nutrients and other measures of "nutrient status." In most cases, energy requirements and vitamin and mineral needs can be met by eating all ration components.

Table 15–8. Vitamins and Mineral Supplements for Cold Weather and Altitude Operations		
Nutrient	**Suggested Amount**	**% DRI**
Vitamin B1, Thiamin	3 mg	200
Vitamin B2, Riboflavin	2 mg	118
Vitamin C	250 mg	417
Vitamin E	400 mg α-TE	1,990
Zinc	15–20 mg	133

Missions at Altitude

Ascent to altitude and flying can cause a variety of disturbances, and adequate nutrition is crucial for maintaining performance. The major nutritional concerns at altitude are:

- Weight loss.
- CHO intake.
- Dehydration.
- Oxidative stress.

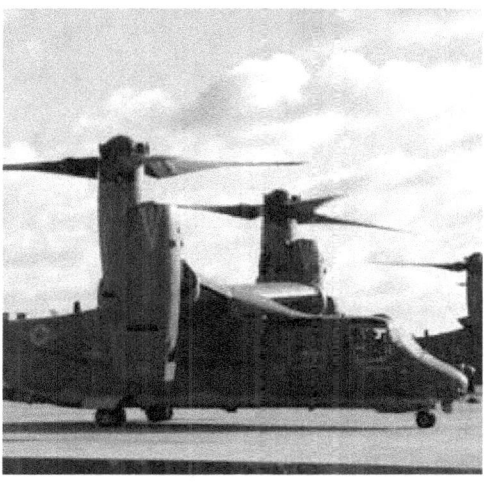

- Nutrition advice for military operations in high-altitude environments.

- A Soldier's Guide to Staying Healthy at High Elevations.

Example:

A WF requires 4,000 kcal/day.

A 50% increase in energy would be = 4,000 x 0.50 or +2,000 kcal

Goal: Eat 5,000 kcal/day

Dehydration in a plane is different from on a mountain.

Weight Loss

Virtually all people who go to high altitudes experience weight loss and loss of lean body mass. At altitudes below 5,000 m weight loss can be prevented by being vigilant about eating on a regular basis. Above 5,000 m, a 5–10% weight loss is inevitable. Energy intakes should range from 3,500–6,000 kcal per day, which is equivalent to eating at least four MREs or two First Strike Rations daily. Some reasons for weight loss at altitude include:

- Increased energy requirements to 115–150% of sea level requirements.

- Decreased sense of taste, which causes a reduction in food intake.

- Changes in the metabolism of fat and CHO.

- Loss of body water from increased breathing rate and dry air.

- Impaired absorption of nutrients.

- Acute Mountain Sickness (AMS), which can cause nausea, vomiting, headache and decreased appetite.

The only way to minimize weight loss is by being vigilant about maintaining energy intake.

Energy requirements may increase 15–50% above requirements at sea level.

CHO Intake

High CHO foods are the preferred energy source at altitude and in flight because they:

- Replete glycogen stores.

- Require less oxygen to produce energy than fat.

- Are the most efficient energy source.

- Can blunt and delay the progression or severity of AMS symptoms (nausea, vomiting, and headache).

- Maintain blood glucose.

Diets should provide at least 400 grams of CHO and CHO should contribute 50–70% of the total energy. This can be accomplished by eating high CHO snacks between meals and drinking CHO-containing beverages during strenuous activity, long flights, and recovery.

Dehydration

Dehydration in a plane is different from on a mountain.

Exposure to high altitude is associated with significant levels of dehydration because water losses are increased. If these losses are not replaced, dehydration will result. Some studies suggest that vigorous hydration may decrease the incidence and severity of AMS. Dehydration will increase the risk of cold injury. The reasons dehydration occurs at altitude include:

- Increased respiratory losses due to increased ventilation.

- Increased urine output due to altitude and cold temperatures.

- Possible diarrheal fluid losses.

- Failure to drink water.

- Poor access to water.

Pilots need to have regular access to a bottle of water or an electrolyte beverage, but on a limited basis. Drinking beverages with sugar is not recommended. Also, coffee, sodas, and teas should be avoided.

Importantly, do not over-exercise before a flight, since strenuous exercise can deplete body water, which may be difficult to replace quickly. Recent illness, fever, diarrhea, or vomiting will also greatly affect the degree of dehydration.

Taking regular sips of cool, 40°F water before feeling thirsty may help prevent dehydration.

Fluid requirements may be > 4 quarts per day at high altitude.

Maintain a drinking schedule and monitor hydration status daily to avoid AMS.

Oxidative Stress

One consequence of altitude exposure is the production of an excessive load of reactive oxygen species. In particular, increased metabolic rate and hypoxic conditions at altitude can increase the production of harmful free radicals. Collective free radicals cause oxidative stress, which may slow blood circulation and impair physical performance. Polyunsaturated fatty acids (PUFAs) are the nutrients most susceptible to oxidative stress. Studies have shown that symptoms of altitude sickness correlate

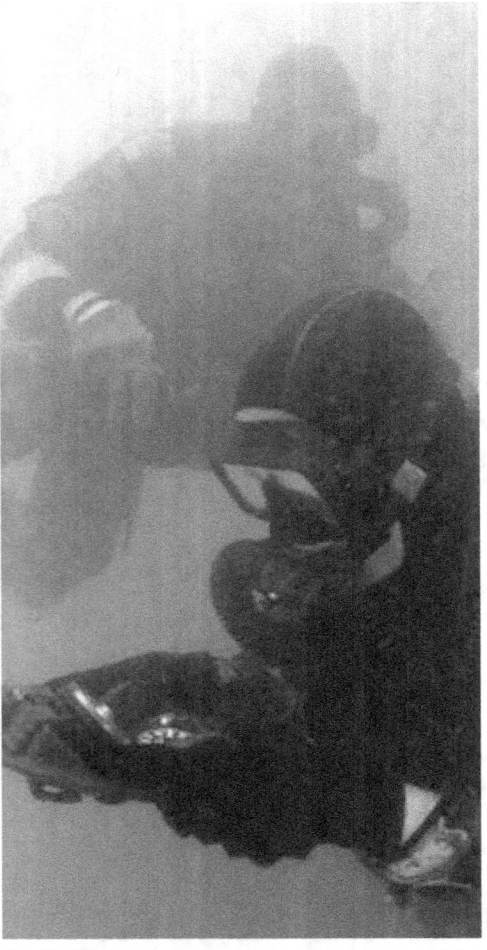

with markers of oxidative stress. Thus, antioxidants have been used to minimize oxidative stress.

Several studies indicate that taking Vitamin E (400 IU/day) may reduce free radical production at altitude, and help maintain blood flow and aerobic energy metabolism in men. Also, a combination of 1,000 mg of Vitamin C, 400 IU of d-α-tocopherol acetate (400 mg α-TE) and 600 mg of alpha-lipoic acid taken in divided doses in the morning and evening was shown to minimize symptoms of altitude sickness and improve energy intake in men. However, the protective benefits of antioxidants against acute mountain sickness are inconsistent.

Although studies are showing benefits of antioxidants, too much may be harmful. Exposure to altitude produces natural adaptations and it is possible that too much of any antioxidant could compromise nature's response to lower oxygen levels. Refer to Table 15-8 for a complete recommendation of vitamin and mineral supplements for cold weather and altitude recommendations.

Missions in Water and at Depth

Like exposure to altitude and cold environments, water operations, especially cold water operations, are associated with increased energy expenditure and marked fluid losses. Thus nutritional concerns for diving are maintaining:

- Energy intake.

- Fluid intake.

- Mineral balance.

- Antioxidant balance.

Energy Intake

When working at the same rate in water as on land, the energy expenditure to accomplish the same task is greater in water. The reasons for this increased energy expenditure during water operations include:

- Greater resistance offered by water.

- Decreased efficiency of movement when thermal protective clothing are worn.

Glycogen stores are rapidly used when performing hard work in cold water. These stores must be replaced between operations to prevent performance decrements. Increasing CHO intake before an anticipated dive has been shown to improve and extend exercise performance during prolonged dives.

Fluid Intake

Immersion in water increases urinary excretion by 2–10 times above normal. Without adequate hydration a diver can quickly become dehydrated and suffer performance decrements. For example, immersion during a single dive for 3 to 6 hours can result in a 2–8 pound loss in body weight by urination; this is equivalent to losing 1–3 quarts of fluid. Importantly, drink fluids with CHO whenever possible to maintain blood glucose. A decline in blood glucose is known to adversely affect performance.

Mineral Balance

Immersion in water, especially cold water, increases urinary losses of magnesium, calcium, zinc, and chromium. It is important to consume foods high in these important minerals to restore immersion-induced losses. See Chapter 4 for foods high in these minerals.

Antioxidant Balance

Like altitude, diving results in greater oxidative stress than working at sea level. This makes sense because with increased depth comes increases in oxygen tension. Oxidative stress is even greater when oxygen is the air breathed at depth. As noted with altitude, some adaptation takes place and natural antioxidant defense systems are "up-regulated" to minimize cell damage from oxidative stress. Despite this, antioxidants have been used to combat potential deleterious effects of oxidative stress. Although no definitive recommendations can be made, some benefits have been noted by taking 1 gram of vitamin C and 400 IU of vitamin E two hours before extended dives. However, a diet high in natural antioxidants should confer protection as well.

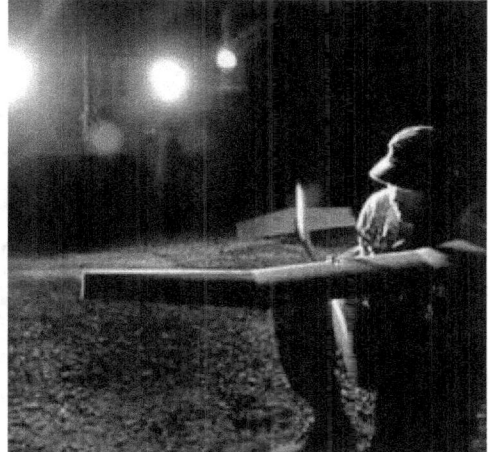

Diving at depth, especially when breathing oxygen-rich gas, facilitates the formation of "reactive" oxygen species.

Mission Scenarios

Nutrition challenges are expected during deployments where harsh environmental conditions, austere living quarters, and lack of food services are the rule. Although nutritional inadequacies can compromise performance, if energy intake can be maintained above 2,000 kcal/day with at least 300 gram of CHO and 60 gram of protein, and fluid status maintained, performance should be sustained over a period of weeks. However, developing sound nutritional plans for training and mission scenarios should help sustain performance. Sample nutrition plans are provided for the following training scenarios:

- Typical Training Day.

- SDV Operation.

- Unconventional Warfare.

- Special Reconnaissance.

- Nighttime Air Mission.

For most scenarios, the macronutrient recommendations assume an energy requirement of 4,000 kcal/day. If energy requirements are lower or higher, the amounts of CHO, protein, and fat should be altered accordingly. **The timing and/or amount of any particular nutrient can be modified to suit individual needs based on the scenario and personal experiences.** Snacks refer to food and beverages that can be carried and consumed while on the mission/operation. Specific foods are not identified, but a list of good field foods, both from rations and commercial off-the-shelf products is included. Each person has individual tastes and it is most important that all food components taken for deployment be tested. The caveat is for extended missions when eating on the economy is the rule, rather than the exception.

Typical Training Day

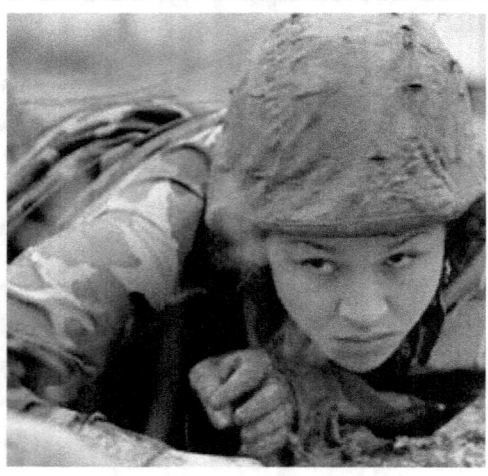

OPORDER:	Get in shape.
Duration:	12 hours.
Chow Availability:	COTS.
Terrain:	Command Dependent.

Nutrition Recommendations:

- Plan a healthy recovery meal after morning PT.

- Maintain a high intake if CHO.

- Drink fluids and eat CHO during long training events.

- Choose plenty of fresh fruits and vegetables, and a variety of whole grains while still on home territory.

Table 15–9. Typical Training Day				
Time	**Activity**	**CHO (g)**	**Protein (g)**	**Fat (g)**
0530	Wake-Up —Juice	50	0	0

Table 15–9. Typical Training Day				
Time	Activity	CHO (g)	Protein (g)	Fat (g)
0630–0830	PT			
0830	Breakfast	100	20	15
0830–1000	Classroom/briefing			
1000–1200	Work on gear/other			
1100	Snack	40	10	6
1300–1330	Break for lunch	120	30	30
1400–1630	10 mile march 2 mile swim 3 hr dive	60	0	0
1630–1730	Clean Gear—snack	40	0	0
1730	End of work day— go home			
1730–1900	Dinner	120	60	40
1900–0530	Personal time and sleep			
2200	Snack	40	10	6
	Total g	570	130	97
	Total kcal	2,280	520	873
	Total Daily kcal	3,673		

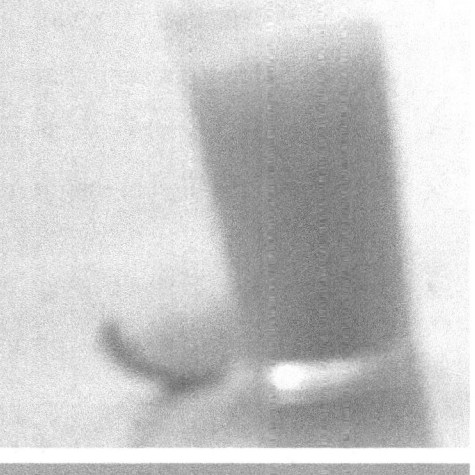

Food Suggestions:

- Yogurt and bagel.

- Whole-wheat crackers.

- Fruit and vegetables.

- Chicken and fish.

- Fruit juices.

- Rice and baked potatoes.

SDV Operation

OPORDER:	Long range insertion.
Duration:	12–14 hours at night.
Chow Availability:	COTS/Rations.
Terrain:	Nautical Environment—Surface water temperature 55–60°.

Nutrition Recommendations:

- Eat a high CHO meal or snack two hours before mission.

- Increase fluids to offset urinary losses.

- Consume CHO rich beverages to maintain blood glucose.

- Consume foods high in magnesium, calcium, zinc and chromium (trail mix, beef jerky).

- Consume a hot CHO beverage upon mission completion, if possible.

- Eat CHO rich foods between sorties.

Table 15–10. SDV Operation				
Time	Activity	CHO (g)	Protein (g)	Fat (g)
1700	Pre-Mission Meal Water 16 oz	100	25	25
1800	Descent 1			
2400	Snack CHO drink, 16 oz	60	10	5
0100	CHO Drink, 32 oz	50	0	0
0200	Descent 2			
0800	CHO Snack Water, 16 oz	60	10	5
0900	CHO drink, 32 oz	40	0	0
1200	Meal Water, 16 oz	100	20	25
1400	Snack Water, 16 oz	60	10	0

Table 15–10. SDV Operation				
Time	Activity	CHO (g)	Protein (g)	Fat (g)
1600–1730	Dinner	100	25	25
	Total g	570	100	85
	Total kcal	2,280	400	765
	Total Daily kcal	3,445		

Food Suggestions (CHO, protein, fat in grams):

- Chunked Chicken and tortilla, 1 serving each—(32, 35, 9).

- Whole-wheat crackers, 10 each—(27, 4, 6).

- Turkey Jerky, 2 oz—(12, 24, 1).

- Soldier Fuel Bar, 1—(40, 10, 9).

- Poppyseed pound cake, 1 piece—(37, 4, 13).

- Fruit nut mix, 0.3 cup—(18, 12, 26).

- Coconut-Almond bar, 1—(56, 16, 12).

- Strawberry-Honey granola, 1 serving—(43, 18, 12).

- Dried cranberries, 0.5 cup—(45, 0, 1).

- Gels, 1 pack—(27, 0, 0).

- CHO Beverage, 8 oz—(15, 0, 0).

Unconventional Warfare

OPORDER:	Train indigenous guerilla force.
Duration:	Multi-year until completion of mission.
Chow Availability:	Limited resupply; be prepared to exist on indigenous, local food sources. Resupplies should include sport bars, CHO-electrolyte packets, and other snacks.
Terrain:	Tropical to sub-artic, with some heavy forested areas.

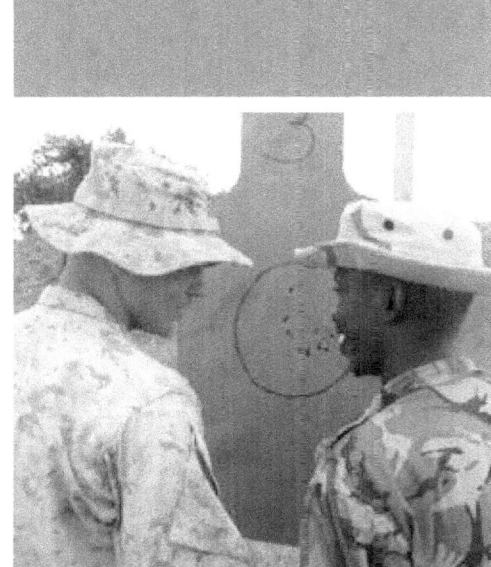

Nutrition Suggestions:

- Purify water.

- Refer to Chapter 14 on Combat Rations and Chapter 13 on Eating Globally.

- Try to maintain 2,000 kcal per day with as much CHO as possible.

- Eat a sport bar every two hours to maintain blood sugar.

- Protein and CHO may come from local sources (animal, legumes, grains, dairy).

- Majority of energy may come from rations (MRE /First Strike Ration) and COTS.

- See section above on hot/cold weather.

Table 15–11. Unconventional Warfare				
Time	Activity	CHO (g)	Protein (g)	Fat (g)
0530	Pre-Mission Meal CHO/PRO beverage	120	10	20
0730	Snack Water, 8–16 oz	40	10	5
0930	Snack Water, 8–16 oz	40	0	0
1130	Lunch Water, 8–16 oz	120	20	20
1430	Snack Water, 8–16 oz	40	10	10
1630	Snack Water, 8–16 oz	120	30	30
1830	Snack CHO/PRO beverage, 8–16 oz	75	10	15
2130	Snack Water, 8–16 oz	40	0	0
Total g		595	90	100
Total kcal		2,380	360	900
Total Daily kcal		3,640		

Food Suggestions (CHO, protein, fat in grams):

- Mountain House Beef Stroganoff, 1 serving—(62, 21, 21).

- Alpine Aire Freeze-Dried Pineapple Chunks, 1 serving—(20, 10, 0).

- Powerbar Endurance sport powder drink, 16 oz—(40, 0, 0).

- Gookinaid ERG drink powder, 8 oz—(40, 0, 0).

- Odwalla Super Protein bars, 1 bar—(31, 16, 5).

- Zapplesauce, 2 serving—(64, 0, 0).

- Carb-BOOM! Gel, 1 pack—(27, 0, 0).

- FSR tortillas, 1 serving—(32, 4, 5).

Special Reconnaissance

OPORDER:	Conduct recon and gain awareness of enemy ground activity.
Duration:	Four cycles of night.
Chow Availability:	Rations/Rations.
Terrain:	Altitude—be prepared to work between 7,000–9,800 feet.

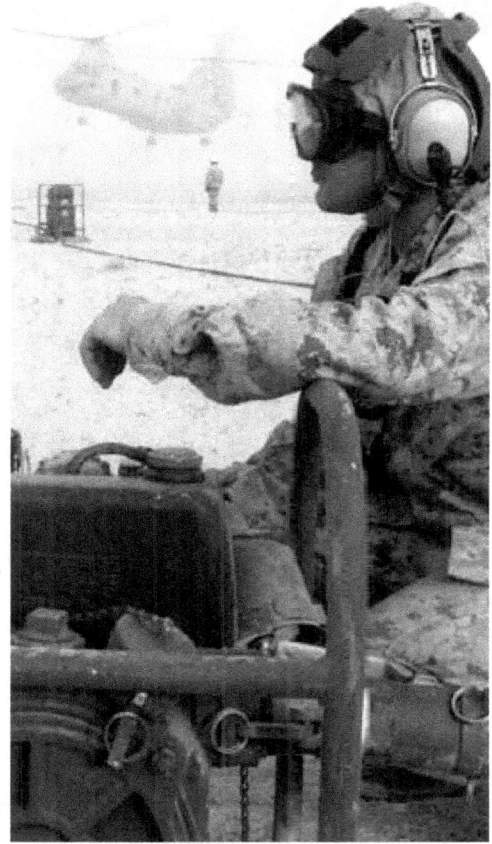

Nutrition Suggestions:

- Pre-mission meal should be high in CHO, protein, and fluids.

- Purify water—hydration critical to minimizing AMS.

- Meals must be easy to prepare, and high in CHO.

- Vitamin E (400 IU) and C (1 gram) may be helpful.

- Moderate caffeine intake may be needed for alertness and cognitive function.

- Easily portable and accessible foods are requisite.

- Minimize fiber intake.

Table 15–12. Special Reconnaissance (SR)			
Time	Activity	CHO (g)	Protein (g)	Fat (g)
1700	Pre-Mission Meal Water, 16 oz	120	40	30
1900				

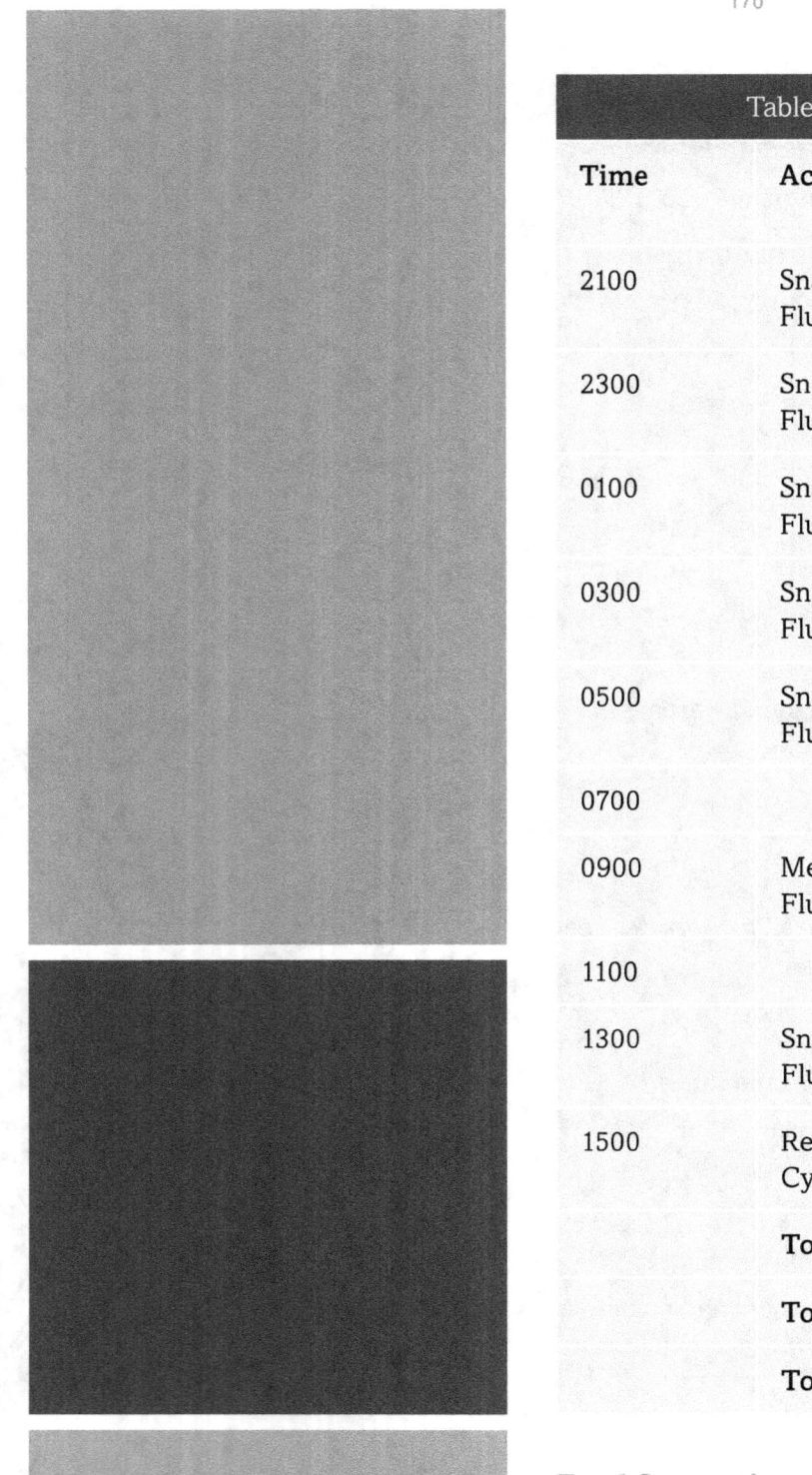

Table 15–12. Special Reconnaissance (SR)

Time	Activity	CHO (g)	Protein (g)	Fat (g)
2100	Snack Fluid, 16 oz	50	0	0
2300	Snack Fluid, 16 oz	40	10	6
0100	Snack Fluid, 16 oz	75	10	15
0300	Snack Fluid, 16 oz	40	10	6
0500	Snack Fluid, 16 oz	40	5	30
0700				
0900	Meal Fluid, 16 oz	100	30	25
1100				
1300	Snack Fluid, 16 oz	40	0	0
1500	Repeat 24 hours Cycle	40	0	0
	Total g	545	105	112
	Total kcal	2,180	420	1,008
	Total Daily kcal	3,608		

Food Suggestions (CHO, protein, fat in grams):

- Beef BBQ pocket sandwich, 1 serving—(40, 9, 9).

- MRE cracker, plain, in FSR—(26, 4, 5).

- HooAH! Cran-Raspberry, 1 serving—(25, 2, 3).

- ERGO drink, 16 oz—(86, 0, 0).

- Zapplesauce, 1 serving—(32, 0, 0).

- French toast pocket, 1 serving—(60, 5, 10).

- Desert Bar, mocha, 1 serving—(21, 2, 15).

- Alpine Aire Freeze-Dried Strawberries, 1 serving—(24, 2, 0).

Nighttime Air Mission

OPORDER: Infiltrate ground troops/bundle drops.

Duration: 10-14 hrs in length.

Chow Availability: COTS/Rations.

Environment: Too hot or too cold during flight, circadian rhythms are periodically switched.

Nutrition Suggestions:

- Plan for a CHO rich pre-mission meal.

- Decrease fluid intake during the mission.

- Consume small, CHO rich snacks on a regular basis to maintain blood glucose.

- Eat a meal after the mission.

- Increase fluid intake after landing to restore fluid balance.

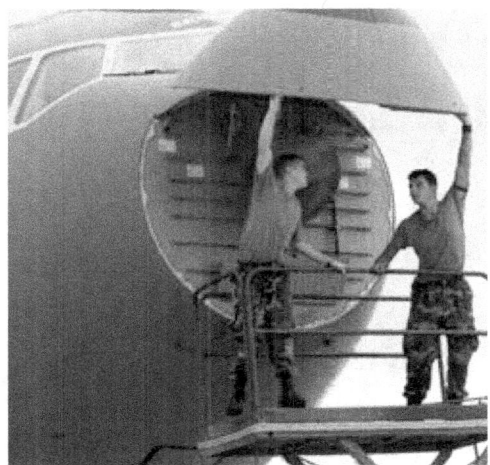

Table 15–13. Nighttime Air Missions				
Time	Activity	CHO (g)	Protein (g)	Fat (g)
1600	Pre-Mission Meal, 8 oz	100	20	20
1900	Snack	40	10	5
2100	Snack	40	10	5
0100	Snack Water, 8 oz	40	0	0
0300	Snack	40	10	10
0500	Snack	40	10	10
0700	Meal Water, 16 oz	100	20	20
0900	**Rest**			
1100		60	5	10

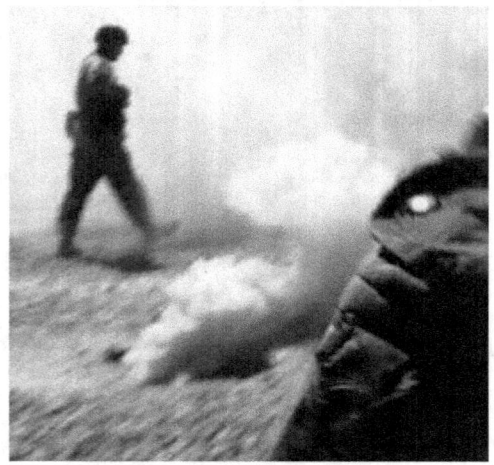

Table 15–13. Nighttime Air Missions				
Time	**Activity**	**CHO (g)**	**Protein (g)**	**Fat (g)**
1300	Snack Water, 8 oz	40	10	5
1500	Repeat Cycle			
	Total g	500	95	85
	Total kcal	8,000	1,520	6,885
	Total Daily kcal	3,145		

Food Suggestions (CHO, protein, fat in grams):

- Mountain House Beef Stew, 1 serving—(54, 36, 16).
- Whole-wheat crackers, 6—(11, 1, 3).
- Beef jerky, teriyaki, 2 oz—(9,11, 4).
- Soldier Fuel bar, 1—(40, 10, 9).
- Zapplesauce, 2—(64, 0, 0).
- Ergo drink, 1—(43, 0, 0).
- Trail mix, 5 oz—(18, 12, 26).
- Box raisins, 1.5 oz—(32, 1, 0).

Summary

The three primary ways to be nutritionally prepared during missions are:

- Eating a high CHO diet to maintain and sustain glycogen stores.
- Being well hydrated—follow a forced fluid replacement schedule since thirst is not a always a good indicator of fluid needs under extreme environmental conditions.
- Eating snacks every 2 hours to maintain blood glucose.

16 Returning to Home Base

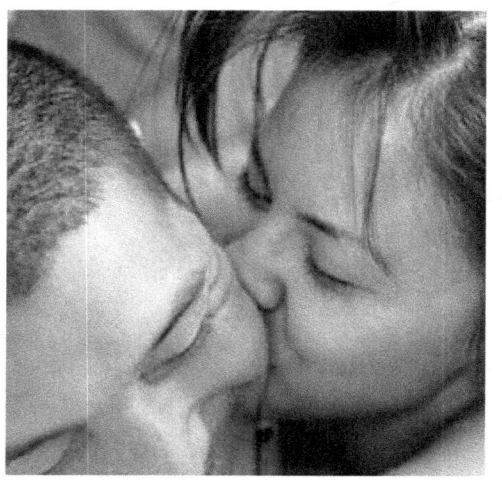

Key Points

- Rest and rejuvenation should be emphasized upon return from deployment to re-optimize mental and physical performance.

- A good night of sleep in a comfortable bed and dark room is essential for recovering from deployments.

- A balanced diet high in complex carbohydrates, such as vegetables, fruit and whole grains, can enhance stress resistance.

- Good nutrition and regular exercise are excellent antidotes to stress.

- Avoid binge eating and drinking upon returning from deployments. Excess food and alcohol intakes can lead to unwanted weight gain and is detrimental to overall health.

Professional athletes have the luxury of going home soon after competition, so life can return to normal. In contrast, Warfighters may be away for extended periods of time and, during those times, can be depleted of essential nutrients needed for health. Choices in food and beverages may be limited in areas without military food service support and local foods may be unsuitable due to sanitation issues. Limited choices can result in significant weight loss. Upon returning home, many will "pig-out" and "drink-like-a-fish," which transforms the warrior athlete into a less than optimal machine. This chapter will provide information about how to regain health and become nutritionally replete upon returning to home base.

The Reality

Many military personnel have expressed concerns about their eating and drinking behaviors upon returning home after a deployment. Stress incurred over the preceding months can sometimes lead to unhealthy decisions that may add greater stress to an already stressful life. Weeks or months away from home can result in feelings of having been deprived of comforts, such as alcohol and favorite foods. This can promote binging on previously unavailable food and beverages. Significant problems, such as weight gain, alcohol dependency, driving under the influence, domestic problems, and even

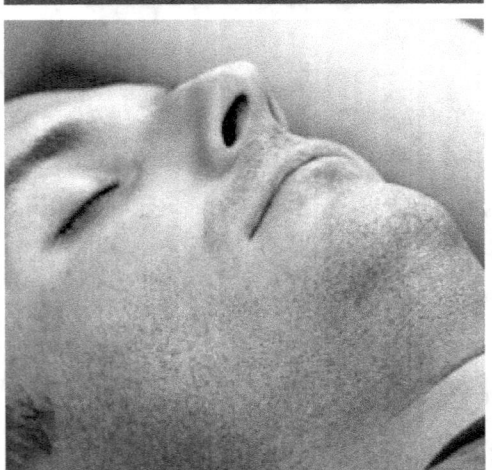

work related conflicts may occur. Choosing good food and making positive lifestyle choices are essential for a smooth transition. Healthy food choices and limiting alcohol consumption will minimize weight increases and help avoid weight fluctuations (gains and losses). Repeated weight loss and/or gain can affect overall military performance and render a finely tuned human vehicle antiquated or useless before its time.

Down Time = Rejuvenation = Reset

Rest is one of the most important aspects of recovery. Mental and physical stressors are common during deployment and resetting the stress-response system is important. Lack of sleep, stress, and inadequate nutrition disrupt the body's finely regulated internal rhythms. Time off upon return from deployment is essential for reconnecting with family, normalizing routines within the household, and resetting internal rhythms.

Sleep

Sleep is vital for re-establishing normal daily rhythms, which are necessary for optimal mental and physical performance. Most hormones, such as the stress hormone, cortisol, and human growth hormone, have day and night cycles: they are greatly affected by loss of sleep. One third of a person's life should be spent sleeping. Most operations away from home allow for minimal sleep, so time at home should ensure high quality, restorative sleep. Sleep is important for:

- Growth and development.

- Restoration of the nervous system.

- Immune function.

- Memory and learning.

- Mood improvement and human behavior.

Sleep is critical—for the brain and the body.

In contrast, chronic lack of sleep increases the risk of developing:

- Obesity.

- Diabetes.

- Cardiovascular disease.

- Opportunistic infections.

- Mood disturbances.

Lack of sleep affects two major body systems: the "master" hormone regulating gland and the autonomic (automatic or involuntary) nervous system. Many factors that control the release of important hormones are regulated during sleep. Also, the signals that usually allow us to be alert and vigilant when awake are maintained in an active state in the absence of sleep. Sleep allows this "sympathetic" nervous system to be reset and restored for the upcoming day. Returning home from deployment is an important time to make sleep a priority. This allows the body to reset biologic rhythms and prepare for repeated military training phases.

Sleeping and feeding are closely related because the hormones regulating appetite (leptin, ghrelin, and insulin) are strongly influenced by the amount of sleep. Sleep deprivation creates an imbalance in the signals for energy balance, and may lead to obesity. According to the Department of Health and Human Services, people who sleep on average, five hours a night are more likely to become obese over time compared to people who sleep seven to eight hours a night. One other potential effect of a continually active nervous system and lack of sleep is the development of glucose intolerance or predisposition to Type II diabetes. This is of utmost concern.

Each menu provides about 1,540 kcals (15% protein, 35% fat, and 50% carbohydrate).

Sleep Disturbers

Factors that may prevent a good night's sleep include:

- **Caffeine**: Receptors that trigger sleep are blocked by caffeine.

- **Nicotine**: May act as a stimulant and decrease ones ability to fall asleep; nicotine withdrawal may cause early awakening.

- **Alcohol**: A sedative that prevents deep, restorative sleep (REM).

- **Pain Relievers**: Most contain caffeine.

- **Exercise**: Daytime exercise may improve sleep, but exercising 1–4 hours before bedtime may cause insomnia.

- **Medications**: Decongestants, steroids and beta-blockers can decrease restorative sleep.

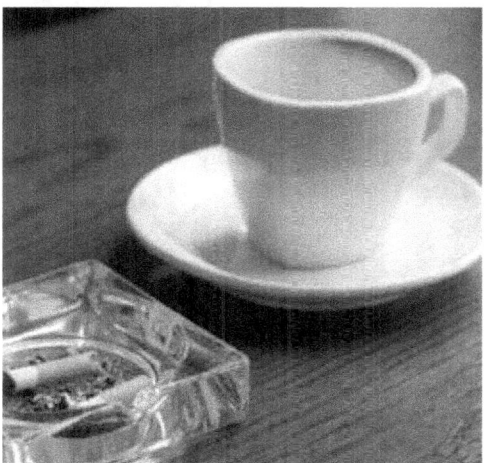

How Much Sleep is Enough?

Every person requires a certain amount of sleep: anywhere from 5–10 hours nightly. Whether a person is getting enough sleep can be determined subjectively from various signs and symptoms. Selected signs of sleep deprivation include:

- Difficulty waking up in the morning.

- Difficulty concentrating.

- Falling asleep during work or class.

- Feelings of irritability, depression, anxiety, and/or moodiness.

Researchers in Australia developed a "sleepiness" scale (Epworth Sleepiness Scale), which is used around the world to measure sleep deprivation. Questions about the likelihood of dozing off in selected situations are asked and the most appropriate answer for each situation is chosen; a score is tallied based on the responses. Total scores are assigned a sleep category ranging from "Enough" to "Severe Sleep Debt."

What is Good Sleep?

Individuals who are tired fall asleep within five minutes or less. Good sleep usually means sleeping in one's own bed, which should be comfortable and quiet. If your partner typically disturbs your sleep, switch to a queen- or king-size bed. Also, try different mattresses and pillows. Other considerations for good sleep include:

- Finding a therapeutic pillow that cradles the neck and allows for sleeping on one's side.

- Making the bedroom a place for sleeping so the body knows the bedroom is a place for rest.

- Making certain the room has adequate airflow and is neither too hot nor too cold.

- Using a fan to block out various noises.

- Hiding the clock so the time and the light can not be seen.

- Making sure the room does not "rise with the sun:" the room needs to be dark in the morning.

Stress

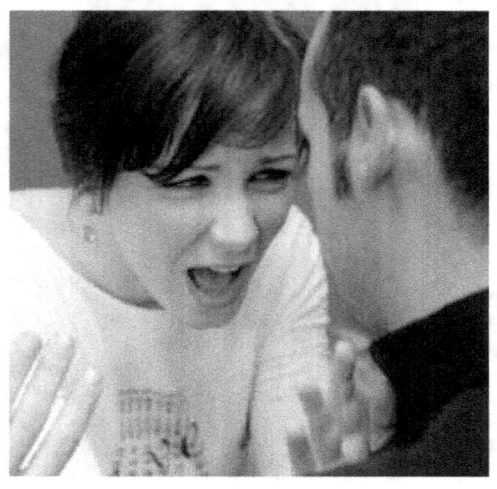

Stress in life is inevitable, and life is all about confronting challenges. The body's two main stress-response systems are the autonomic nervous system (discussed above) and the hypothalamic-pituitary adrenal (HPA) axis. Chronic stress can disrupt the regulation of these two systems. For example, lack of sleep can affect hormones like cortisol and growth hormone, among others.

Dealing with stress when returning home is not easy. Loved ones at home have not had the same experiences. Loved ones may feel stressed as well, and overly stressed people are not always attentive. Everyone perceives their particular stressors as very important, and there is no way to change this perception. What is clear is that the stress of war, which is considered an extreme stress, can lead to violent, abusive or threatening behaviors. Upon return from war, alcohol and other drugs are often used to reduce stress, but, in reality, they create more stress. It is also important to realize that overly stressed people are more likely to smoke, have poor dietary habits, and be physically inactive.

Warfighters are mentally and physically resilient individuals, and most are likely to experience Post-Traumatic Stress Growth (PTSG), rather than PTSD. PTSG implies inner growth and increased determination—unlike PTSD. Nevertheless, conversations with team members and other Warfighters about deployment experiences are healthy and can be cathartic. Military commands have embedded operational, combat-focused psychologists who are familiar with unit missions, demands, and lifestyles; these persons are available to speak with military personnel at any time. They can inspire and promote PTSG. In addition, Family Services are available on Navy, Marine Corps, Army, and Air Force bases. These services provide resources for stress management, improving relationships, money management, and referrals to help resolve family and personal issues. Such resources are invaluable upon re-entry after deployment.

Diet, Exercise, and Stress Connections

Research continues to show a strong relationship between nutrition and stress, and exercise and stress. A high-fat, high-sugar diet in combination with chronic stress are major factors in the development of obesity. In contrast, selecting a diet rich in complex carbohydrates, such as colorful vegetables, fruits, and whole grains, can help enhance stress resistance. Upon returning home, if body weight is 10–15 pounds lower than pre-deployment, it is easy to feel comfortable selecting "comfort" foods (high-fat/high-sugar), but before long, weight creeps back up and exceeds what is optimal for missions. Making wise diet and exercise choices will promote a more rapid readjustment.

Anti-Stress Diet

An anti-stress diet will do wonders upon returning home. It is becoming clear that stress can lead to obesity because of the stress hormone cortisol. Eating an anti-stress diet means resisting an increase in body fat, which typically accumulates in a man's belly. Products and foods to avoid for minimizing stress on the body include:

- Caffeine.

- Hard liquor.

- Tobacco.

- Trans-fats from fried foods, red meats, and highly processed foods.

Essential nutrients are important in combating stress. These include the minerals, zinc and magnesium, and vitamins C, B, and E. The B vitamins and magnesium are involved in the production of serotonin, which helps

Good nutrition and regular exercise are excellent antidotes to stress.

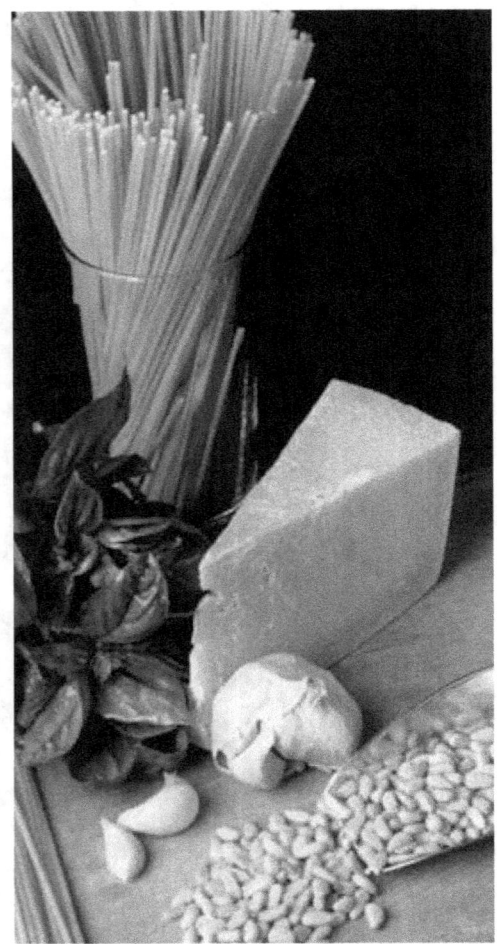

regulate mood and relieve stress. Foods high in these nutrients are the foods of choice. If one had to develop a list of foods important for countering stress, many whole foods would be on the list. Table 16–1 provides a list of foods that will help alleviate or prevent some of the consequences of chronic stress. In addition, these foods will help minimize weight gain due to overeating and excess intake of high-fat, high-sugar foods. If 90% of the foods selected can be from the list of nutrient dense foods, the other 10% can be from "comfort foods."

Sudden weight gain due to overeating and excessive alcohol consumption will compromise performance and health.

Table 16–1. Top Foods for Combating Stress	
Almonds	Green tea, herb teas, lemon water
Sweet potatoes, beets	Broccoli, zucchini, green beans
Whole-grain rice or pasta	Sushi
Goat Cheese, whey	Carrots, tomatoes, peas
Cantaloupe, other melons	Salmon, other cold water fish
Blueberries, kiwi, grapes	Garlic

Exercise

Physical exercise is one of the most effective ways of relieving stress. The act of physical exertion causes the body to release chemical substances (endorphins) similar in nature to opiates. These natural substances make us feel good and have no adverse effects, unlike many other drugs. Regular exercise should be a scheduled part of any returning home plan— it may be in the form of enjoyable recreational activities, such as camping, hiking, basketball, surfing, cycling, or running and weight lifting. Making room for exercise will help keep life issues under control and promote relaxation.

Exercise will also prevent belly bulge and deconditioning.

Meal Planning Strategies for Special Gatherings

The key to avoid gaining excess pounds is to make smart selections at parties. The rule "it is not a good idea to shop at the commissary while hungry" applies to parties; do not attend a party on an empty stomach. The following strategies can help maintain nutritional balance, while still having a good time:

- Eat a regular meal before the event to avoid overeating.

- Eat breakfast to control hunger and avoid the tendency to overeat.

- Drink water to avoid dehydration, and minimize hangover symptoms, from alcoholic beverages: one glass of water should be drunk for every glass of alcohol consumed.

- Focus on appetizers: variety in selection and appropriate portion size are key.

- Resist deep-fried appetizers: stock the plate with shrimp and vegetables.

- Resist cream based soup, cheese-filled dishes, pies, pastries, and many baked goods.

- Choose fruits and vegetables, as well as whole grain breads and crackers, that are high in dietary fiber. They will curb appetite, taste great and add vitamins and minerals.

- Choose sweets made with dark chocolate. A small amount of dark chocolate can be healthy and satisfying.

- Drink sparkling apple juice or cider, seltzer mixed with fruit juices, flavored calorie-free water and/or low-sodium vegetable juice to maintain hydration and avoid a hangover.

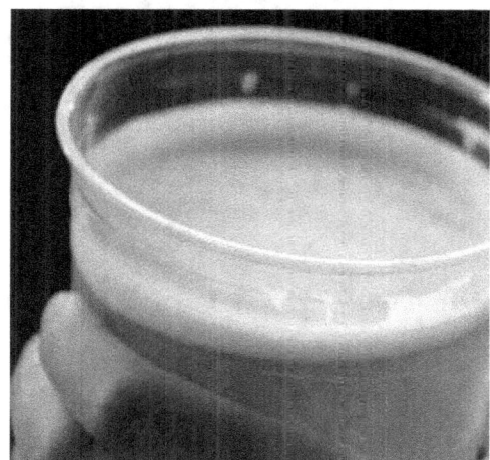

Alcohol

At least 23% of service members admit to drinking heavily—a statistic that hasn't been lowered in over 25 years. Alcohol-related incidents (DUI, drunk and disorderly, alcohol related reckless driving, sexual assaults, suicidal attempts) continue to rise at alarming rates, and teams have been formed to assess what is being done and what should be done to address the problem. A 2007 report from the Department of Defense Task Force on Mental Health noted a three-fold increase in alcohol-related incidents from the third quarter of FY 2005 to the third quarter of FY2006. Unfortunately, no noticeable increases in persons entering the alcohol program accompanied the rise in incidents. In fact, only 41% of Warfighters involved in alcohol-related incidents were referred to the alcohol program.

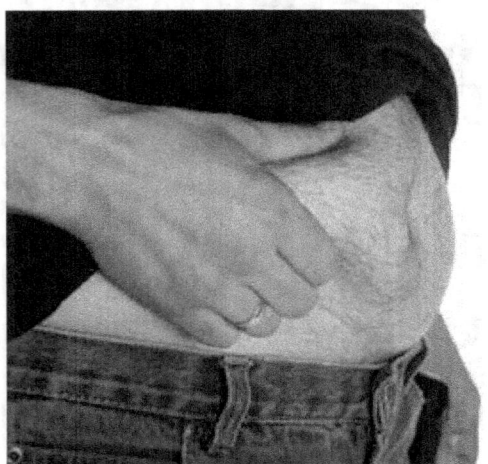

In addition to alcohol-related incidents, alcohol contributes to obesity and belly fat. Alcohol provides 7 kcal per gram of empty calories—its nutrient density is low. The liver processes alcohol, which is why many alcoholics and heavy drinkers experience liver damage.

Alcohol abuse is a problem and returning home from deployment is a critical time for abuse to surface.

How Much Alcohol is Enough?

Two servings are considered moderate. **One** serving consists of:

- A 12-oz bottle or can of beer.

- A 5-oz glass of wine.

- A shot of liquor or spirits (either straight or in a mixed drink).

Calories from alcohol tend to be stored in the abdomen as belly fat.

"For many people, moderate drinking is probably safe. It may even have health benefits, including reducing your risk of certain heart problems. Anything more than moderate drinking can be risky. Binge drinking—drinking more than five drinks at a time—can damage your health and increase your risk for accidents, injuries, or assault."

—National Institute on Alcohol Abuse and Alcoholism

It is recognized that alcohol (wine) in moderation (two drinks a day for men) increases good cholesterol (HDL). However, beyond these amounts, alcohol has many harmful effects, and moderation requires forethought and discipline.

Binge Drinking

Binge drinking is a sign of being overstressed.

Binge drinking is drinking until intoxicated over a period of at least two days. Being repeatedly intoxicated overrides participation in usual activities and fulfillment of other obligations. According to results from the Army's "Self Reported Health Risk Appraisal" of 404,966 soldiers, "those consuming more than 21 drinks per week were at six times the risk for subsequent alcohol-related hospitalizations."

Relationships and internal rhythms will be seriously compromised if alcohol is substituted for good food, performance, and health.

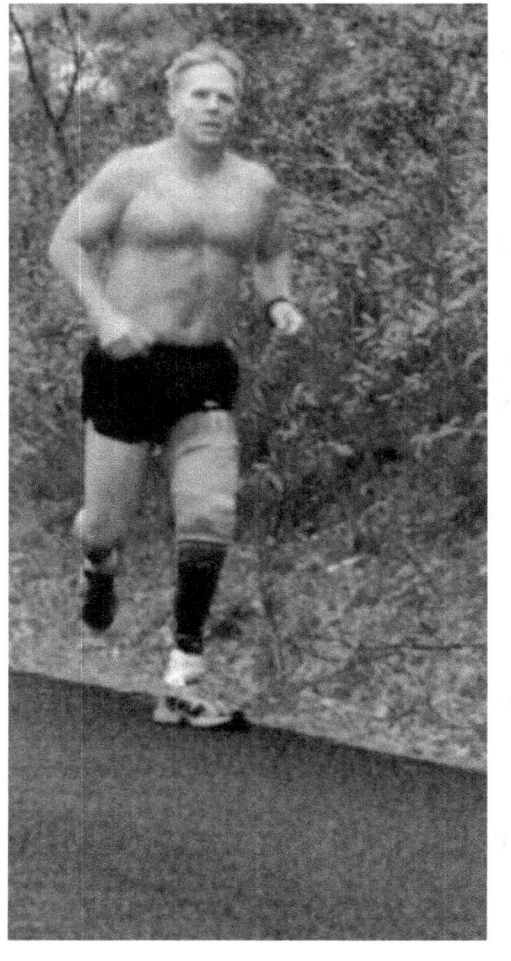

17 The High Mileage Warrior Athlete

Key Points

- Try to maintain weight minimize weight cycling—multiple episodes of weight loss.

- Pain from arthritis can be reduced by choosing healthy foods and foods high in anti-inflammatory compounds.

- NSAIDs should be used on a very limited basis.

- Foods, not supplements, should be the primary source of nutrients. Food is the best and cheapest way to take in essential nutrients.

- The risks of developing hypertension, coronary heart disease, diabetes, and cancer increase with age. Eating the right type of foods can limit risk factors associated with these chronic diseases.

The aging warrior athlete is concerned about general health. Punishment from years of heavy physical activity can take a toll on Warfighters. This chapter will look at various diseases associated with aging and what can be done to promote good health into retirement. Major health problems can include arthritis, musculoskeletal injuries, weight gain, hypertension, coronary heart disease, Type II diabetes, metabolic syndromes, and cancer. Each will be briefly discussed.

Dietary Approaches for the High Mileage Warfighter

Many foods, or dietary components, contain biologically active substances that may confer health benefits or desirable physiological effects beyond basic nutrition. Such foods are now called "functional foods." Knowing which foods contain these important components allows greater control of personal health through food choices. Foods that impart specific health benefits include fruits and vegetables, whole grains, fortified or enhanced foods and beverages. The health-promoting attributes of many traditional foods are being discovered, and new food products with beneficial components are being developed. Selected functions served by food components would include:

Table 17–1. Examples of Functional Food Classes
Carbohydrates
Carotenoids
Fiber
Flavonoids
Isocyothionates
Minerals
Phenolic Acids
Phytoestrogens
Plant Sterols
Prebiotics
Probiotics
Vitamins

- Restoring fluid balance.
- Improving endurance.
- Enhancing muscle strength.
- Preventing muscle/joint injuries or fatigue.
- Enhancing immune function.
- Preventing heart disease and diabetes.
- Preventing high blood pressure.
- Reducing pain and inflammation.

Dependence on Vitamin M (Ibuprofen)

Ibuprofen is a non-steroidal anti-inflammatory drug (NSAID) used to relieve pain, fever, and inflammation. It is commonly known as Vitamin M among the military community because of its frequent use. Some Warfighters are known to take up to 2 grams/day. The use of ibuprofen is not without risks. Common side effects include gastrointestinal distress, raised liver enzymes, salt and fluid retention, and hypertension. The risk of myocardial infarction appears to be higher among chronic users of ibuprofen than non-users.

Some foods or food components can serve as alternatives to NSAIDs (see Chapter 12 for a list of these products). The alternatives are both dietary and exercise oriented. Table 17–2 presents a list of products that are recognized for providing pain relief. Some can be taken as foods rather than supplements.

Table 17–2. Anti-Inflammatory Foods and Dietary Supplements	
Substances	**Significant Sources**
Glucosamine	No food sources. Dietary supplements are derived from hard outer shells of shrimp, lobsters, and crabs.
Chondroitin	No food sources. Dietary supplements sources are derived from shark and beef cartilage or cow trachea.
Vitamin E	Poultry, seafood, vegetable oils, wheat germ, fish oils, whole-grain breads, fortified cereals, nuts and seeds, dried beans, green leafy vegetables, fruits, and eggs.

Table 17–2. Anti-Inflammatory Foods and Dietary Supplements	
Substances	**Significant Sources**
Selenium	Tuna, wheat germ, garlic, whole grains, sunflower seeds, eggs, and Brazil nuts.
Omega-3 Fatty Acids	Cold water fish (salmon, mackerel, sardines, and herring), flaxseed, soybeans, soybean oil, pumpkin seeds, and walnuts.
Capsaicin Cream (from chili peppers)	Pharmacies and health food stores.
Bioquercitin	Apples, yellow and red onions, cherries, certain citrus fruits, leafy vegetables, broccoli, raspberries, black tea, green tea, red wine, and red grapes.
Methylsufonyl-methane or MSM	Onions, garlic, and cruciferous vegetables, such as cabbage and broccoli.

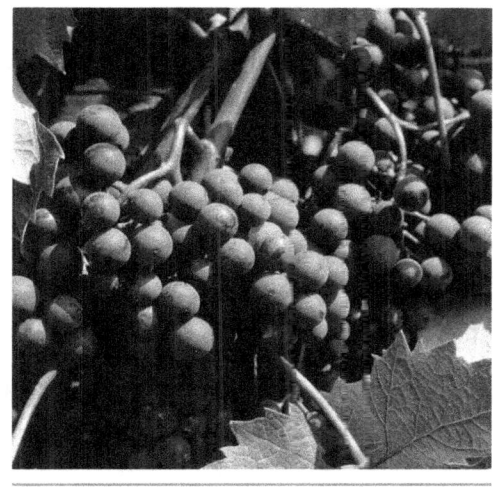

Dietary sources of antioxidants are superior to single or combined antioxidant supplements.

Antioxidants

Oxidation, or the production of free radicals, is a normal consequence of strenuous exercise, exposure to UV-radiation, pollutants, chemicals, and extreme environments, and just living. Usually the body's natural defense systems, or "antioxidants" can neutralize free radicals and render them harmless. However, the body can be overwhelmed by free radicals, which may result in structural and functional damage. Inflammation, infection and muscle injury from exercise may reflect an inability to defend against oxidant stress. In addition, free radical damage contributes to aging and a host of illnesses, including cancer and heart disease.

People who chew tobacco should make sure their diets are high in antioxidants.

A well-balanced diet providing many antioxidant-rich foods supports the body's natural defense against free radical threats and protects against tissue damage. Importantly, more than 4,000 compounds in foods act as antioxidants. These could also be considered functional foods. The most well known antioxidants are vitamins C and E, beta carotene and the mineral, selenium. However, those are only a few of the many substances.

> Coenzyme Q10 is sold as a dietary supplement, but the FDA does not "approve" dietary supplements for effectiveness.

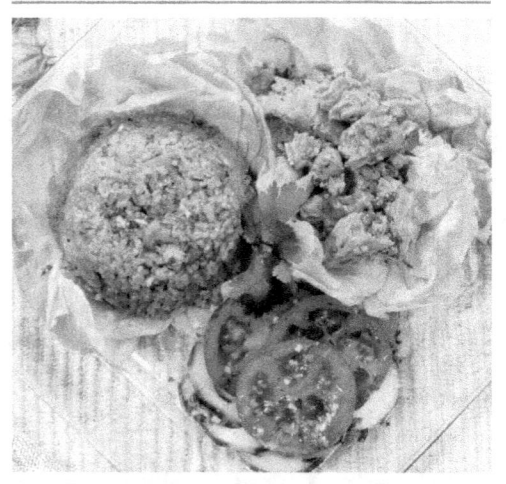

Coenzyme Q10

Coenzyme Q10 (also known as ubiquinone or CoQ10) is a vitamin-like substance made by the body. It is essential for producing the energy (ATP) that makes cell function. Tissue levels of CoQ10 decrease with age and are low in some chronic diseases (heart, cancer, diabetes, hypertension). Physician sometimes prescribe CoQ10 to increase tissue levels, but the effectiveness of CoQ10 is not definitive. However, it appears to help with mild hypertension.

It is also important to note that statins inhibit the body's ability to make CoQ10. Some health care providers request that Warfighters taking statins should also take CoQ10. This should be done under the guidance of a physician and at the appropriate dose.

A Well-Balanced Diet

A well-balanced diet of fruits, grains, and vegetables will provide the requisite antioxidants and other nutrients. Many studies have shown that people who eat a well-balanced diet are less at risk for developing many chronic diseases.

> Eat at least 4 servings of fruit and 5 servings of vegetables daily.

Arthritis and Musculoskeletal Injuries

About one-third of U.S. veterans suffer from some form of arthritis, which may be due to orthopedic injuries sustained on active duty. Also, musculoskeletal injuries are the leading cause of medical profiles for active duty personnel. This rate is double that seen in non-veterans. Because military training imposes a significant risk for musculoskeletal injuries, it may be inevitable that Warfighters are likely to develop some form of arthritis. However, the pain can be minimized by choosing foods high in various nutrients.

Osteoarthritis

Rates of osteoarthritis are on the rise within the military. Osteoarthritis, which occurs when cartilage in the joint deteriorates, can be extremely painful. Being overweight is a major risk factor for osteoarthritis, so weight loss may relieve some of the joint pain. Another approach to pain reduction is low-impact exercise. Moderate cardiovascular exercise and strength training will improve physical performance and reduce pain.

Treatment

Traditional methods, such as prescription drugs and surgery, are available to relieve discomfort and improve mobility but these approaches will not lead to a cure. Alternative therapies include dietary manipulations. Consuming foods high in anti-inflammatory substances (green vegetables, carrots, avocados, pecans, soy products, brown rice, millet, oats, wheat, and barley, sesame, flax, and pumpkin seeds) and cold-water fish (salmon, sardines, herring, and tuna), and minimizing dietary intake of alcohol, coffee, sugar, and hydrogenated fats (margarine).

Two popular supplements for arthritis and musculoskeletal injuries are glucosamine and chondroitin sulfate. They are widely used and prescribed, but more information is needed to determine the best dose and form.

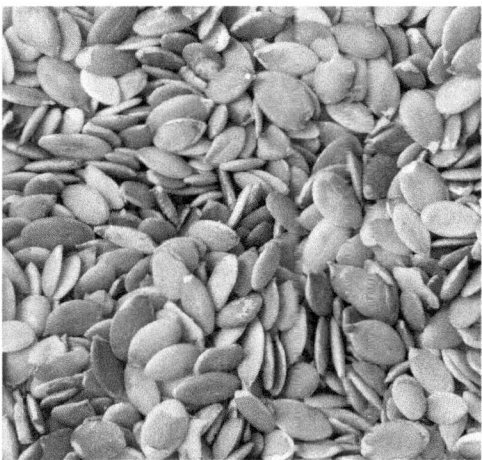

Weight Gain and Weight Maintenance

As the warrior ages, it is easy to increase body weight and difficult to take it off. Food quality, sleep hygiene, and portion control are very important issues for maintaining the desired body weight.

Food Quality

The quality of food is especially important for high mileage Warfighters. Decreasing the amount of "junk food" in the diet is essential as you age. "Junk" foods not only add chemicals and processed food fillers to the body, but also empty calories. Eating sweets and highly processed foods, like potato chips, store purchased baked goods, and alcohol, deplete the body of high performance catalysts needed for other functions. They also add toxins to a healthy, fine-tuned body.

Quality of Sleep

There is more to weight gain than food and exercise. Sleep habits can negatively affect body weight. Adequate rest is essential when possible. The fewer hours slept, the higher the chance of being overweight.

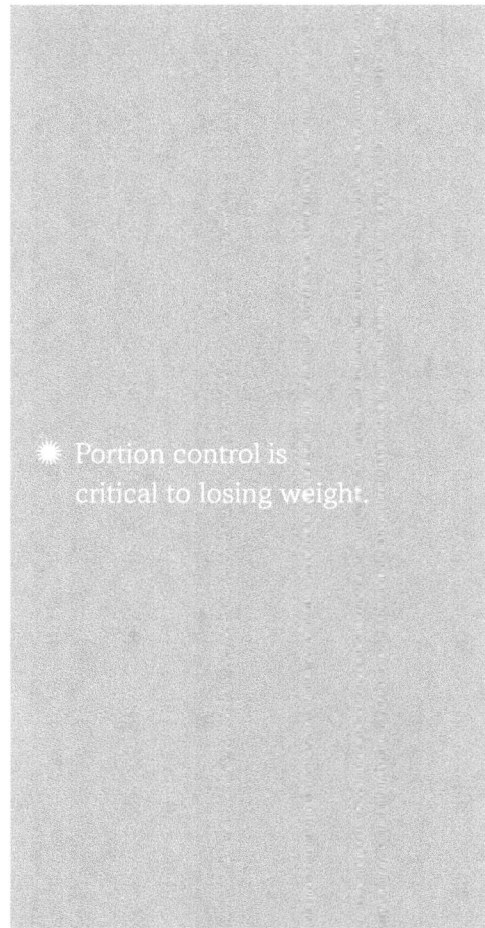

✳ Portion control is critical to losing weight.

Preventive Measures

- Increase sleep, when possible.

- Count and contain the number of "Happy Hour" drinks consumed.

- Keep up the cardio workouts—focus on long, slow, distance training for better fat utilization.

- Combine cardio and strength training at least three times a week.

Weight Loss

As discussed in Chapter 2, energy intake and energy expenditure must be balanced to maintain weight. Weight loss can be made easy following this principle: less "junk" foods and more exercise equal weight loss, right? Yes and no. In the ideal world this would work, but numerous life variables, like parties, social drinking, and binge eating, get in the way. See Chapter 2 for tips on how to make weight loss a part of every day life are provided

Yo-Yo Dieting

Yo-yo dieting, or weight cycling, is defined as repeated weight loss by repeated dieting and, when more food is introduced, subsequent regaining of weight. Repeated weight gains and losses can cause health problems. As a Warfighter, dieting may not be a major issue, except when returning home. Once home, binge eating and drinking often occur, which can result in a rapid weight gain (see Chapter 16).

High Blood Pressure, or Hypertension

High blood pressure, or hypertension, is the most common "heart" condition among active duty personnel. The major behaviors to consider when trying to lower or prevent high blood pressure include:

- Keeping a healthy weight: as little as a 5-10% weight loss can drop blood pressure significantly.

- Being moderately physically active every day of the week, if possible.

- Eating a healthy diet.

- Avoiding foods high in sodium.

- Drinking alcoholic beverages in moderation.

Blood pressure is measured as two numbers—systolic (heart contracts) over diastolic (heart relaxes) pressure. Normal blood pressure values are less than 120 (systolic) and 80 (diastolic) mm Hg. Values higher than 120 and 80 may be a problem and should be discussed with a physician.

If you are at risk for hypertension, the Dietary Approaches to Stop Hypertension (DASH) eating plan is the diet most often recommended. In brief, the plan suggests the following:

• Eating more fruits, vegetables, and low-fat dairy foods.

• Cutting back on foods high in saturated fat, cholesterol, and total fat.

• Eating more whole grain products, fish, poultry, and nuts.

• Eating less red meat and sweets.

• Eating foods rich in magnesium, potassium, and calcium.

• Reducing sodium (salt) to 1,500 mg a day (about $^2/_3$ teaspoon).

A healthy, well-balanced diet is more than fueling muscles; it also protects the heart.

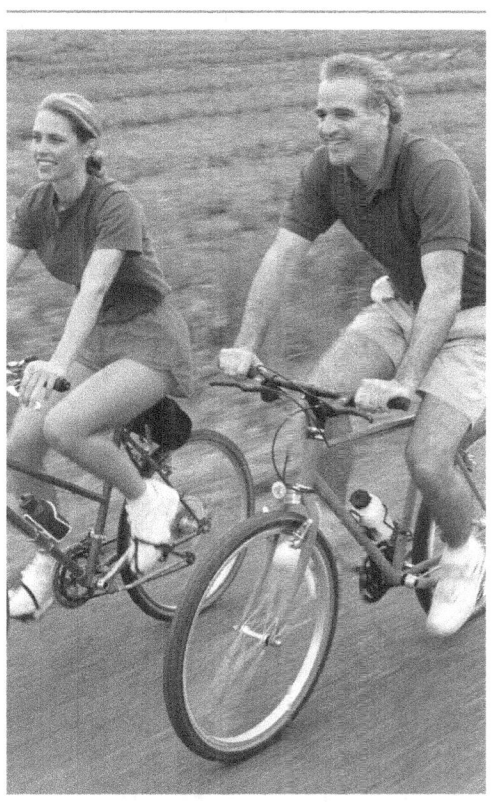

Coronary Heart Disease (CHD)

The high mileage warrior athlete is not invincible from coronary heart disease (CHD). Age naturally increases the risk, if diet is neglected. Maintaining good eating patterns and cardiovascular fitness can decrease the high mileage warrior's chance of developing CHD.

Eating fruit, vegetables and whole grains is a good place to start. Dietary guidelines from the American Heart Association are provided below.

Building Blocks for Life	
Healthy Eating Patterns	**Healthy Body Weight**
• Eat a variety of fresh fruits and vegetables.	• Balance energy needs.
• Eat whole grain pastas and rice.	• Physical activity.
• Select low-fat products.	• Avoid the "Apple Shape" body.
	• Waist girth needs to be below 40".
Desirable Blood Lipid Profiles	**Desirable Blood Pressure**
• Limit use of saturated fats.	• Limit use of salt.
• Avoid trans fats.	• Limit alcoholic consumption (2 for a day).
• Replace saturated fats with fats from vegetables, fish, and nuts.	• Maintain body weight.
	• Follow DASH Diet.

Table 17–3. Risk Factors for CHD
Diabetes
Cholesterol (HDL/LDL)
High Blood Pressure
Smoking/ Tobacco Use
Alcohol Consumption
Family History of Heart Disease

Eating a variety of fish
can improve lipid levels!

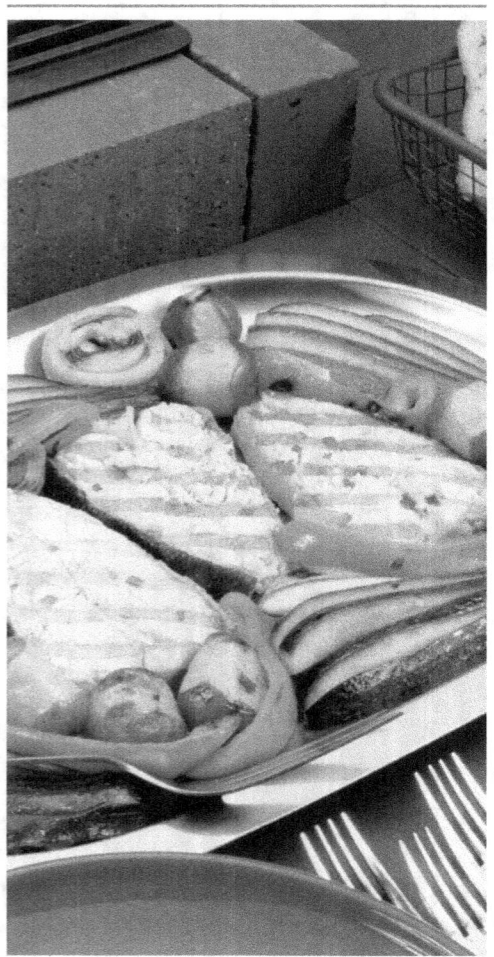

Lowering Risks

The risk of CHD can be lowered, but some factors cannot be controlled:

- Age.

- Gender: Men have an increased risk of developing heart disease.

- Family history of cardiovascular disease or diabetes.

Luckily, there are some factors for which you do have control. They include the following:

- Diet.

- Exercise patterns.

- Annual checkups.

- Frequent blood pressure screenings.

- Smoking history.

- Lipid profile.

Lipid Profiles

A lipid profile is a panel of tests used to determine the risk of CHD. The test measures levels of Total Cholesterol, High-Density Lipoprotein Cholesterol (HDL or good cholesterol), Low-Density Lipoprotein (LDL or bad cholesterol) and triglycerides in blood. Physicians use the results (in combination with other known risk factors) to develop a treatment plan, which should be treated seriously, and to assess the effectiveness of the plan.

Treatments for High Risk Lipid Profiles

Three easy treatments for reducing high risk lipid profiles include:

- Change your diet.

- Exercise regularly (aerobic exercise).

- Quit smoking.

Nutritional Choices to Protect Your Heart

The easiest way to protect the heart is by choosing foods known to be effective in reducing the risk of CHD. Some foods known to decrease the risk of developing CHD are presented in Tables 17–4 and 17–5..

Table 17–4. Heart Healthy Foods	
Soy	Isoflavones compounds in soy products may reduce LDL ("bad") cholesterol. Enjoy foods such as tofu, soy nuts, soy flour, and enriched soymilk.
Beans	Eating a cup of beans daily, no matter which kind, can lower cholesterol by 10% in six weeks.
Salmon	Omega-3 fatty acids—found in salmon and other cold-water fish—help lower LDL ("bad"), raise "good" HDL cholesterol, and lower triglycerides.
Avocado	A great source of heart-healthy monounsaturated fat that may help raise HDL ("good") and lower LDL ("bad") cholesterol levels.
Garlic	Garlic helps stop artery-clogging plaque from forming at its earliest stage by keeping individual cholesterol particles from sticking to artery walls.
Spinach	A daily ½ cup of spinach, which is rich in lutein, guards against heart attacks by helping artery walls "sluff off" cholesterol that causes clogging.
Walnuts, Cashews and Almonds	These nuts have all been linked to healthy hearts and contain vitamin E, monounsaturated fats, and magnesium.
Tea	Antioxidants in green tea lower total cholesterol levels and improve the ratio of HDL ("good") to LDL ("bad") cholesterol.
Dark or Bittersweet Chocolate	The flavonoids in dark chocolate help keep blood platelets from sticking together and may even help keep arteries unclogged.

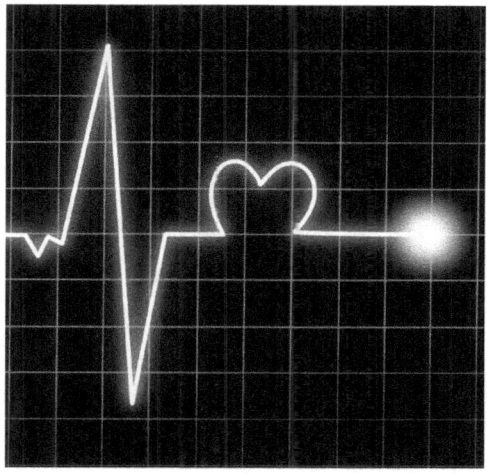

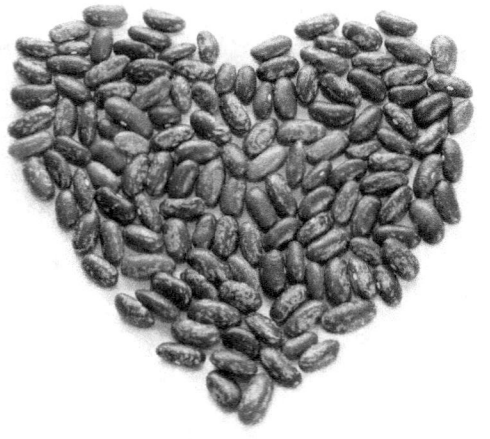

Table 17–5. Nutrients that Protect the Heart		
Nutrient	**Foods**	**Risks Reduced**
Soluble fiber	Oats, oat bran, barley, rye, flax seed, legumes, psyllium husk, dried fruits, apples, pears, citrus fruit, carrots, nuts, dried beans, and peas.	Helps lower blood cholesterol.
Omega-3 fatty acids	Cold water fish, such as salmon, halibut, scallops, tuna, mackerel, cod, shrimp, snapper, and sardines, and vegetables such as flaxseeds, pumpkin seeds, sesame seeds, walnuts, soybeans, dried cloves, cauliflower, mustard seeds, boiled cabbage, broccoli, romaine lettuce, spinach, dried oregano, tofu, brussels sprouts, green beans, strawberries, and turnip greens.	Lowers blood pressure and triglycerides; helps prevent clot formation and irregular heart beats; defends against inflammation.
Vitamin B6	Beans, nuts, legumes, eggs, meats, fish, whole grains, and fortified breads, and cereals.	A deficiency of any will increase homocysteine levels, which is associated with risk of coronary heart disease.
Vitamin B12	Eggs, meat, poultry, shellfish and milk products.	
Folate	Fortified grains, leafy green vegetables, legumes, seeds, and liver.	
Vitamin E	Wheat germ, corn, nuts, seeds, olives, vegetable oils (corn, sunflower, soybean, cottonseed), spinach and other green leafy vegetables, and asparagus.	Limits LDL oxidation and slows down plaque formation.

Drug Treatments to Improve Lipid Profiles

Many physicians prescribe pharmaceutical agents to improve lipid profiles, because they are highly effective. Table 17–6 provides a snapshot of drugs prescribed to Warfighters, with an emphasis on statins. Some people who take statins develop exercise-related rhabdomyolysis, or muscle breakdown, which can be dangerous. Physicians may recommend taking Coenzyme Q10 in combination with statins, but evidence to support this is lacking. However, taking 50 mg daily of a USP approved Coenzyme Q10 supplement cannot hurt and may be helpful, particularly if there is a family history of high cholesterol levels.

Table 17–6. Classes and Types of Drugs to Improve Lipid Profiles		
Class	**Type**	**Expected Result**
Resin	Cholestyramine (Questran) and Coestipol (Colestid).	• Lowers cholesterol by binding bile acids in gastro-intestinal tract.
Triglyceride-lowering Drugs	Fibrates (Lopid or Tricor, nicotinic acid).	• Reduces triglyceride production and removes it from circulation. • Increases HDL levels.
Statins	Fluvastatin (Lescol), Lovastatin (Mevacor), Simvastatin (Zocor), Pravastatin (Pravachol), Atorvastatin (Lipitor).	• Reduce production of cholesterol in liver. • Reduces LDL by up to 40%. • Helps reduce size of plaques on artery walls.

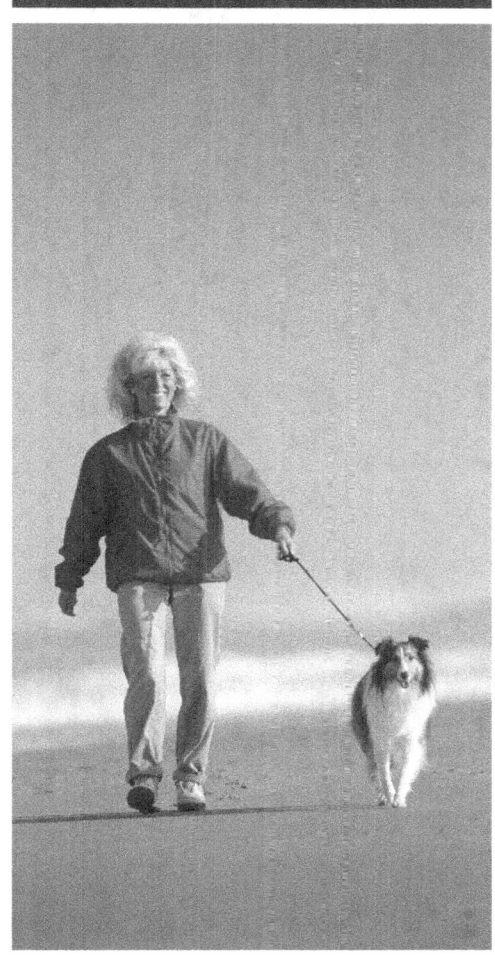

Some research shows that persons taking statins and consuming foods high in omega-3 fatty acids have a better chance of avoiding heart problems than those who took only statins. Again, eating foods high in omega-3 fatty acids may help protect against heart disease.

The primary food sources of omega-3 fatty acids are the oils from some fish and plants. Cold-water fish, such as salmon, mackerel, halibut, sardines, and herring, are rich sources. Plants that contain oils with omega-3 fatty acids include flaxseeds, soybeans, pumpkin seeds, and walnuts. New Zealand green lipped mussels are also an excellent source of omega-3 fatty acids.

Type II diabetes, which is closely related to obesity and physical inactivity, can be controlled by diet and regular exercise.

Type II Diabetes

The incidence of Type II diabetes among adults in the military has risen markedly in the last decade, and is expected to double in the next 50 years. Those with diabetes are twice as likely to develop cardiovascular problems than those who are not diabetic. The prevalence of Type II diabetes among high mileage Warfighters is unknown, but certainly of concern because if undiagnosed and untreated, the risk of developing other chronic diseases increases.

Metabolic Syndrome

Metabolic Syndrome, a disorder of the 21st century, is brought on by a sedentary lifestyle, stress, poor dietary choices (fast foods and highly processed foods), and other unhealthy lifestyle choices. About 10 years ago, before we understood the various contributing factors, this constellation of factors (which occur together) was called "Syndrome X." Now it is clearly recognized as Metabolic Syndrome. In particular, belly fat or central adiposity is present. "Central obesity" is determined by measuring waist circumference: a man with a waist circumference $\geq$ 37 inches (94 cm) is considered at risk. However, for Metabolic Syndrome to be diagnosed, at least two of the following other factors must also be present:

- Serum triglyceride levels are $\geq$150 mg/dl or being treated for this lipid problem.

- Serum HDL cholesterol levels are < 40 mg/dl.

- Systolic blood pressure is $\geq$130 or diastolic blood pressure is $\geq$85 mmHg or being treated for high blood pressure.

- Fasting plasma glucose concentration is $\geq$100 mg/dl or a diagnosis of Type II diabetes has been made.

If you think you have one or more of these "factors" you should consulted your doctor about having metabolic syndrome.

Some foods may inhibit cancer development.

Cancer

Various factors contribute to the development of cancer: genetics, immune function, environment, and diet. A Mediterranean diet, fiber rich diets, and other diets high in colorful fruits and vegetables, protect against cancer. In contrast, a high alcohol intake, with the exception of moderate consumption of wine, has been associated with promoting some cancers. Wine appears to lower the risk of several chronic diseases, perhaps because of the high phytonutrient and antioxidant levels.

18 Sustaining Health for the Long-Term Warfighter

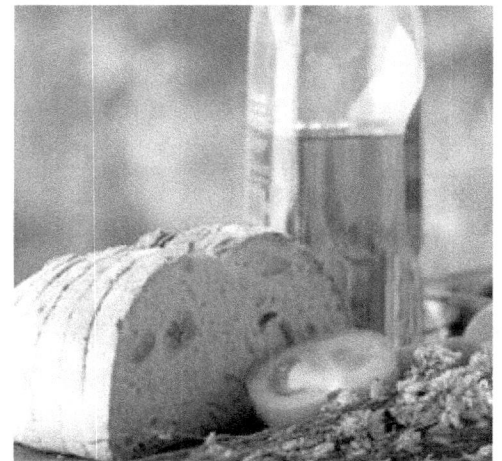

Key Points

- Eating a variety of foods is one key to healthy living.

- A Mediterranean Diet has been shown to confer a long, healthy life.

- Healthy bones require adequate calcium intake and regular physical activity.

- Eating many different colorful real foods, which contain important protective compounds—phytonutrients, promote life-long health.

- At least 3–5 servings of colorful vegetables, 2 or more servings of fruit, and 6 or more servings of whole grain products, should be consumed per day, whenever possible.

- Products containing probiotics (yogurt, kefir, sauerkraut) may be helpful for maintaining a healthy digestive tract.

- Alkaline-forming, rather than acid-forming, foods are important during periods of high stress.

It is possible to be a Long-Term Warfighter if good habits are developed at a young age and sustained throughout life. These "good" habits include a nutritious diet and a balanced exercise program If good habits are developed, the risks of developing musculoskeletal injuries and many other chronic diseases associated with aging will be minimized. This chapter discusses the proper dietary plan to maintain a healthy life.

Principles of Good Eating

- Variety.

- Balance.

- Moderation.

A variety of foods must be consumed to obtain all the requisite nutrients for a strong, healthy body. Eating the same foods is not only boring, but decreases the opportunity to include diverse nutrients in your diet; it can also mean taking in the many environmental pesticides and chemicals on

A healthy diet is achieved by balancing a variety of foods from the major foods groups.

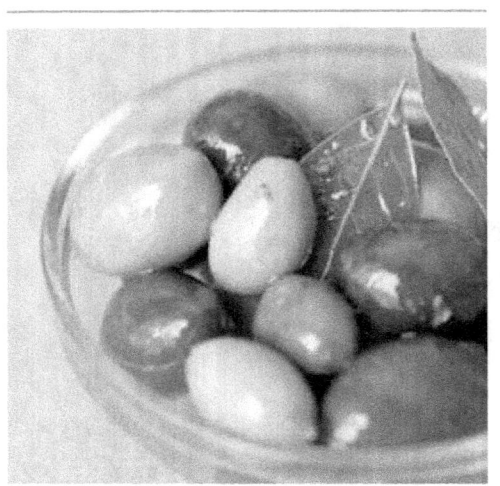

those particular foods. For example, some fish are tainted with mercury, so eating the same kind of fish daily could result in accumulation of mercury. Likewise, if strawberries were the only fruit eaten, the body would accumulate the pesticides from the strawberries. In addition, the nutrients potentially derived from eating a variety of foods would be limited. Fresh and dried fruits, fresh vegetables, whole grains, nuts, eggs, dairy products, meats, poultry, and fish are all nutritious: they provide a ready supply of energy and nutrients to keep the body healthy.

Moderation is perhaps the most difficult goal to achieve without planning meals and snacks in advance. If one meal contains high-fat foods, another meal needs to be low in fat. Advance planning allows all foods to be eaten without incurring an energy deficit or surplus.

90% of your foods should be healthy. Limit junk food to only 10% of your diet.

Mediterranean Diet

One diet singled out as healthy for all ages is the Mediterranean Diet. Research has shown that this type of diet, which is higher in monounsaturated fats than other diets, results in lower blood sugar and cholesterol levels and lower blood pressure than a typical American diet. This is attributed to using olive oil (a monounsaturated fat), consuming lots of fruits and vegetables, and also drinking some red wine. Grapes used to make the wine contain powerful antioxidants.

There is not an official "Mediterranean" diet because at least 16 countries border the Mediterranean Sea and not all of the same foods are eaten. However, there are similarities to the dietary patterns. They include:

- High intake of fresh fruits, vegetables, bread, wheat and cereals, potatoes, beans, nuts and seeds.

- Weekly intake of up to 4 eggs.

- Minimal intake of red meat.

- Low to moderate intake of dairy products, fish, and poultry.

- Frequent and regular use of olive oil.

- Low to moderate intake of red wine.

Omega-3 Fatty Acids

Omega-3 fatty acids were discussed in Chapter 3, but more information on these "polyunsaturated" fatty acids (PUFA) is important because of their health benefits. The important omega-3 fatty acids are alpha linolenic acid (ALA), eicosapentaenoic acid (EPA), and docosahexaenoic acid (DHA). The body cannot make these "fats," but interconversions with omega-6 fatty acids can occur. For example, vegetarians rely on the conversion of ALA into EPA and DHA.

Fish and seafood, particularly oily fish (sardines, salmon, trout, mackerel, herring, and anchovies) are excellent sources of omega-3s. Green vegetables and some nuts and seeds (tofu and other forms of soybeans, canola and soybean oils, walnuts, brazil nuts, and flaxseed) are sources of ALA. Flaxseed (linseed) oil is the best concentrated source of ALA.

A low dietary intake of omega-3 fatty acids has been associated with heart disease, stroke, cancer, inflammatory conditions and auto-immune diseases, and possibly negative mood, depression and other mental health conditions. Thus, a diet that provides adequate amounts of omega-3 fatty acids is important.

How Much is Needed?

Although the exact amount of omega-3s needed for optimal health is unknown, intakes $\geq$ 650 mg/day, or 0.3% of total calories, for EPA and DHA have been recommended. The recommended intake of ALA is 1.6 grams/day for men. An omega-3 deficiency is nonexistent in healthy individuals. Table 18–1 below provides the EPA and DHA content of various foods sources. Clearly, eating 3 ounces of tuna (or the like) each day provides the recommended amounts of omega-3s. Table 18–2 provides the ALA content of various plant products. Eating less than 1 oz of walnuts provides more than the amount recommended.

Diets of today are often high in saturated and trans fatty acids (discussed in Chapter 3), and low in omega-3 fatty acids. The ratio of omega-6 to omega-3 fatty acids in the diet today ranges from 14:1 to about 20:1. A healthier ratio would be 5:1. It should be noted that food sources of omega-6 fatty acids in the diet are ample: omega-6 are found in margarines and vegetable oils.

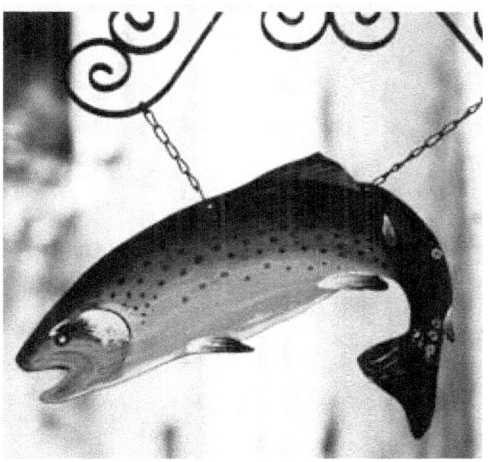

Table 18–1. Content of EPA and DHA in Various Fish Products				
Fish (3 oz)	EPA (mg)	DHA (mg)	Total EPA+ DHA (g)	Total Fat (g)
Bass, Striped	184	637	0.8	2.5

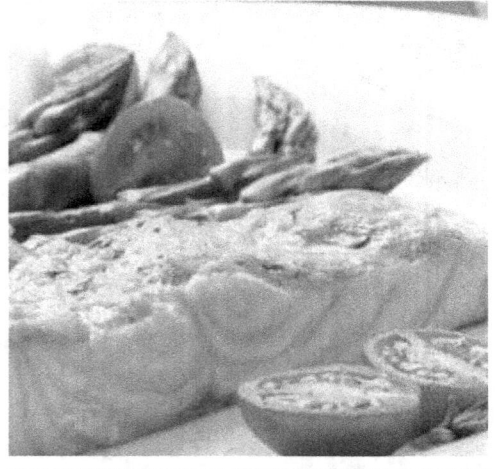

Table 18–1. Content of EPA and DHA in Various Fish Products				
Fish (3 oz)	EPA (mg)	DHA (mg)	Total EPA+ DHA (g)	Total Fat (g)
Catfish, farmed	42	109	0.2	6.8
Clams (9 small)	117	124	0.2	1.1
Fish sticks (~3 sticks)	126	212	0.3	11.1
Flounder & sole	207	219	0.4	1.3
Haddock	65	138	0.2	0.8
Halibut	77	318	0.4	2.5
Herring, Kippered	825	1,003	1.8	10.5
Mackerel, Pacific	555	1,016	1.6	8.6
Mackerel, Atlantic	428	594	1.0	15.1
Oysters, Eastern, wild, raw (~6)	228	248	0.5	2.1
Perch, Atlantic	88	230	0.3	1.8
Rockfish	154	223	0.4	1.1
Salmon, Atlantic, farmed	587	1,238	1.8	10.5
Salmon, Atlantic, wild	349	1,215	1.5	6.9
Salmon, Coho, farmed	347	740	1.1	7.0
Salmon, Sockeye, canned, drained	418	564	1.0	6.2
Salmon, Coho, wild	341	559	0.9	3.1
Sardines, Pacific, packed in tomato sauce	520	845	1.4	1.2
Sardines, Atlantic, oil-packed	402	432	0.8	9.1
Swordfish	111	579	0.1	4.4
Trout, Rainbow, farmed	284	697	1.0	6.1

Table 18–1. Content of EPA and DHA in Various Fish Products				
Fish (3 oz)	EPA (mg)	DHA (mg)	Total EPA+ DHA (g)	Total Fat (g)
Trout, Rainbow, wild	398	442	0.8	4.9
Tuna, Bluefin	309	910	1.3	5.3
Tuna, White, water-packed, drained	198	535	0.1	2.5
Tuna, Light, water-packed, drained	40	190	0.2	0.7
Tuna, Light, oil-packed, drained	23	86	0.1	7.0

Eat a variety of fish at least twice a week and include other foods rich in ALA.

Table 18–2. ALA Content of Various Vegetable Products		
Vegetable/Nuts/ Seeds (3 oz)	ALA (mg)	Total Fat (g)
Brazil Nuts	30	56.5
Flaxseeds	19,400	35.8
Soybeans, green, boiled	301	5.4
Spinach, raw	56	0.13
Sunflower seeds, dry roasted	59	42.3
Tofu	495	7.4
Walnuts, English	7,700	55.5
Winter Squash	31	0.12

Source: United States Department of Agriculture: National Nutrient Database for Standard Reference, Release 19 (http://www.nal.usda.gov/fnic/foodcomp/search/). EPA and DHA values not available for all foods.

Increasing omega-3 intake through foods is preferable to supplements.

Despite being a rich source of omega-3 fatty acids, fish and seafood are potentially major sources of environmental contaminants. Thus, fish con-

sumption is an example where the potential benefits and risks may be in competition. However, it is still acknowledged that the health benefits of eating fish outweigh the risks.

Fish Oil Supplements

Because many people do not like or do not have access to foods high in omega-3s, fish oil supplements are commonly taken. However, fish oil supplements should only be taken under the care of a physician. The most common side effect of fish oil supplements, which was discussed in Chapter 11, is gastrointestinal complaints. It is also possible high intakes of omega-3 fatty acids (> 3 grams/day) may result in prolonged bleeding time.

See www.usp.org for USP-approved fish oils.

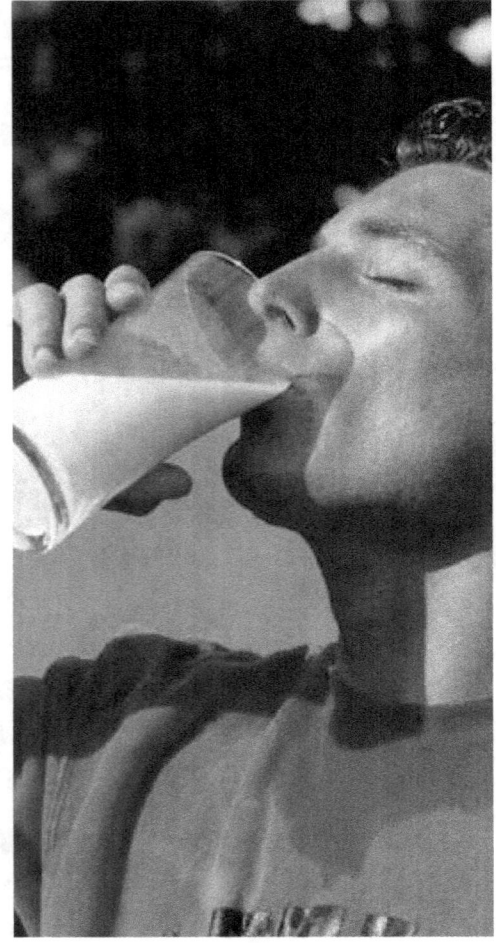

Bone Health

The health status of bones is determined by various lifestyle behaviors between birth and age 30. Bone health is of great concern in military training because stress fractures can eliminate potential "wannabe's" from the playing field. The major determinants of achieving "peak bone mass" during adolescence and early adult life are diet and physical activity.

The primary nutrients for achieving healthy bones are calcium, vitamin D, protein, and other essential minerals. Calcium is one of the most abundant minerals in the body, yet one frequently lacking in the diet of all individuals. On average, daily intake of calcium ranges from 500–700 mg, which is much lower than the suggested level of 1000 mg.

Milk, milk products, and calcium-fortified products are important to bone health. An inadequate intake of calcium can lead to borrowing calcium "reserves" from the bones to meet the body's needs; with a prolonged deficit, osteopenia or low bone mass may develop. A list of foods with high calcium and vitamin D content is presented below. Note that non-fat milk products have a higher calcium content than their low- or full-fat counterparts.

Table 18–3. Foods with High Calcium and Vitamin D Content		
Food	**Amount**	**Calcium Content (mg)**
Yogurt, plain, non-fat	8 oz	450
Yogurt, plain, low-fat	8 oz	350–415

Table 18–3. Foods with High Calcium and Vitamin D Content		
Food	**Amount**	**Calcium Content (mg)**
Yogurt, low-fat, with fruit	8 oz	250–350
Milk, skim	1 cup	302–316
Milk, 2%	1 cup	313
Cheddar cheese	1 oz	204
Provolone cheese	1 oz	214
Mozzarella cheese, part skim	1 oz	207
Ricotta cheese, part skim	1 cup	337
Swiss cheese	1 oz	272
Almonds	½ cup	173
Figs, dried	10 figs	269
Orange juice, calcium fortified	1 cup	250
Orange	1 medium	56
Rhubarb, cooked with sugar	½ cup	174
Collards, turnip greens, spinach, cooked	1 cup	200–270
Broccoli, cooked	1 cup	178
Oatmeal, with milk	1 cup	313
Salmon, canned, with bones	3 ½ oz	230
Sardines, canned, with bones	3 ½ oz	350
Halibut	Half fillet	95

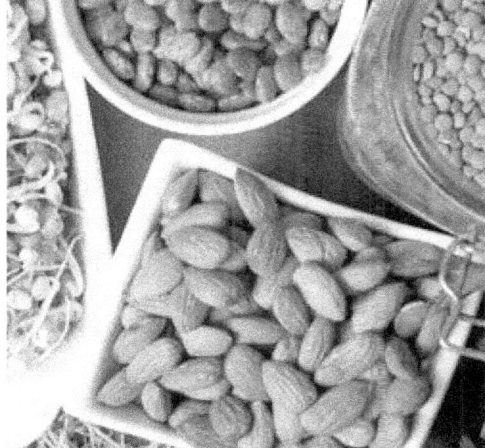
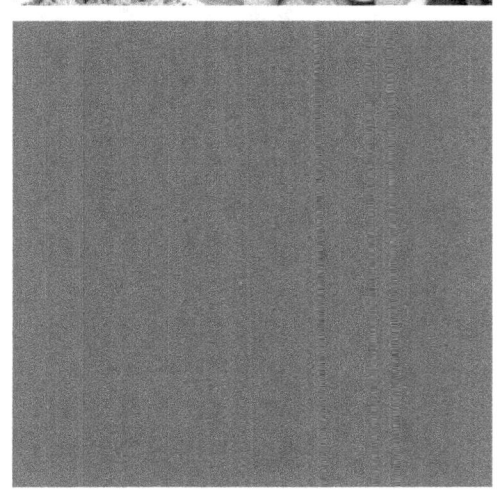

One of the primary reasons for a low dietary intake of calcium is that sodas and colas have replaced milk as the beverage of choice: on average, 23 gallons of milk are consumed per person per year as compared to 49 gallons of soft drinks. Not only have soft drinks replaced milk as the beverage of choice with meals, but they also contain phosphoric acid, which may disturb the natural balance of bone growth. Cola soft drinks are especially harmful due to the caffeine content. Caffeine may interfere with the absorption of calcium from foods and/or supplements, and compromise bone mineral density.

Other reasons why bone health is not what it should be relates to physical activity patterns. Many young men of today are sedentary—playing video games may maintain healthy bones in the fingers and hands, but regular, weight-bearing aerobic exercise and an active lifestyle are essential for promoting good bone health. Other dietary and lifestyle patterns that may compromise bone health include:

- \> 3 alcoholic beverages/day.
- An acidic diet.
- Smoking/smokeless tobacco.
- Excessive intakes of Vitamin A (i.e., retinol).
- Excessive intakes of protein.

Stress Fractures

It is not uncommon for Warfighters to develop stress fractures, which is a consequence of poor bone health and physical fitness. Risk factors for stress fractures include:

- Short height.
- Low bone density or poor bone structure.
- Smoking.
- Alcohol consumption.
- Low calcium intake.
- Low fitness and/or activity levels before enlistment.
- Previous injury.
- Poor muscle strength.

However, in addition to the risk factors noted above, several aspects of military training may contribute as well. These include:

- Training schedules with too much, too soon.
- High running mileage.
- Excessive loss of calcium in sweat.
- Boot/shoe fitting and design.

Phytonutrients

One reason the Mediterranean diet is so healthy is because most of the foods provide phytonutrients (phytochemicals). Phytonutrients are substances found in plants that protect against bacteria, viruses, and fungi. Eating a variety of many colorful foods that contain phytochemicals (fruits and vegetables, whole grains, cereals, and beans) appears to decrease the risk of developing certain cancers, diabetes, hypertension, and heart disease. The actions of phytonutrients vary by color and type of food: they may act as antioxidants, anti-inflammatory agents, and/or other nutrient protectors. Table 18–4 below provides a partial list of phytonutrients and food sources of these important nutrients. Phytonutrients may also be considered functional foods, as discussed in Chapter 17.

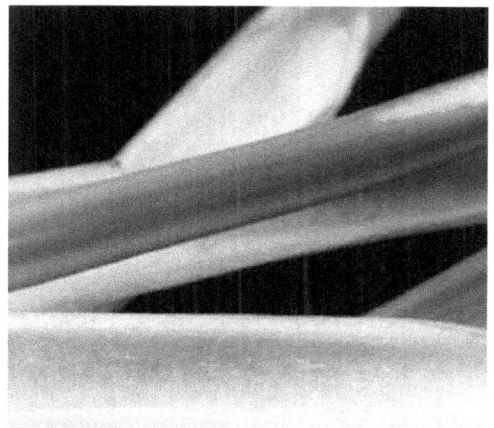
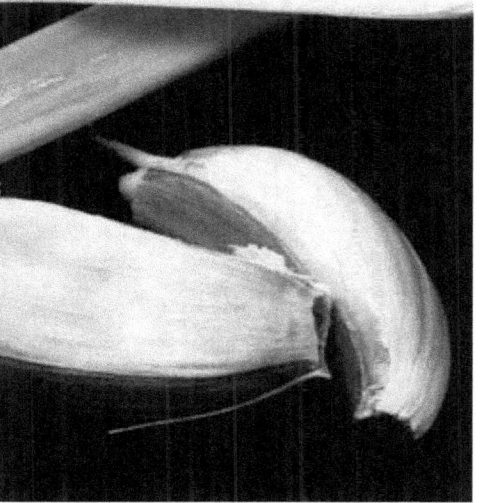

Table 18–4. Types of Phytonutrients and Good Food Sources	
Phytonutrients	**Sources**
Allicin	Onion, garlic
Anthocyanins	Red and blue fruits (raspberries, cranberries, cherries, and blueberries) and vegetables.
Bioflavonoids	Citrus fruits.
Carotenoids	Dark yellow, orange, and deep green fruits and vegetables (tomatoes, parsley, oranges, pink grapefruit, and spinach).
Flavonoids	Fruits, vegetables, wine, green tea, onions, apples, kale, and beans.
Indoles	Bok choy, cabbage, kale, brussels sprouts, and turnips (cruciferous vegetables).
Isoflavones	Soybeans and soybean products.
Lignins	Flaxseed and whole grain products.
Lutein	Leafy green vegetables.
Lycopene	Tomato products.

Phytonutrients should be derived from real foods, **not** dietary supplements.

Table 18–4. Types of Phytonutrients and Good Food Sources	
Phytonutrients	**Sources**
Phenolics	Citrus fruits, fruit juices, cereals, legumes, and oilseeds.

At present, a recommended daily allowance for phytonutrients does not exist. However, eating a variety of foods, including plenty of fruits and vegetables, will ensure an adequate intake. Phytonutrients are now being added to supplements, but it is most likely that their healthful effects are due to their natural packaging. Other foods high in phytonutrients include the following:

Broccoli	Berries	Soynuts	Pears	Turnips
Celery	Carrots	Spinach	Olives	Tomatoes
Lentils	Cantaloupe	Garlic	Apricots	Onions
Seeds	Soybeans	Green Tea	Apples	Cabbage
Brussels Sprouts	Bok Choy	Kale	Red Wine	Grapes

Dietary Fiber

Dietary fiber is a critical component of the diet for health. However, during missions and operational scenarios when performance is critical to the end result, dietary fiber may need to assume a back-seat role.

What is Dietary Fiber?

Dietary fibers, non-starch forms of carbohydrate obtained from plants, are structural components that cannot be digested by the body. Some types of dietary fiber are cellulose, dextrins, inulin, lignin, chitins, and pectins. Because dietary fiber is neither digested nor absorbed, it is not a nutrient like vitamins, minerals, protein, fats, and carbohydrates, but it is still an essential part of a healthy diet.

Insoluble Fiber verses Soluble Fiber

Dietary fibers are classified as soluble or insoluble, and most fiber-rich foods contain some of both types. These two types function differently in the body. Insoluble fibers, the predominant fiber in most foods, absorb water in the gastrointestinal tract and promote regular elimination of stools.

Dietary Fiber:

A form of carbohydrate that is not classified as a nutrient and it cannot be digested.

Insoluble Fiber:

Absorbs water in the gastrointestinal tract and promote regular elimination of stools.

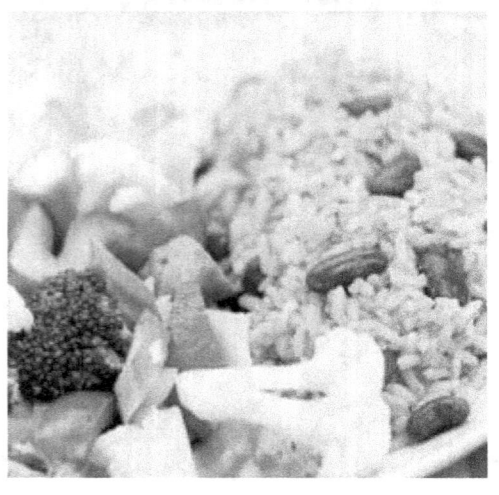

An increase in stool weight and a faster time for meals to be digested and eliminated are common for diets high in insoluble fiber are ingested. In contrast, soluble fibers undergo processing to yield compounds that confer health benefits. For example, soluble fibers such as oat bran appear to lower serum cholesterol and help regulate blood sugar levels.

These special effects of dietary fiber have prompted many health agencies to make specific recommendations regarding how much dietary fiber a diet should provide.

Eat More Fiber

The National Cancer Institute, the American Heart Association, the National Academy of Sciences, and the United States Department of Agriculture all have dietary recommendations for fiber because of its role in reducing the risk factor for various chronic diseases:

- Gastrointestinal diseases.
- Hypertension.
- Diabetes.
- Heart disease.
- Several types of cancer, including colon cancer.

In contrast, a high-fiber intake is associated with a decreased risk. For these reasons, increasing your intake of dietary fiber may be very important with respect to your future health. Recommendations for intake of dietary fiber include:

- Consuming at least 3–5 servings of various vegetables, 2 or more servings of fruit, and 6 or more servings of grain products
- Taking in between 20–35 grams of dietary fiber per day.

The first recommendation is easy to follow because their typical serving is likely a quarter of a Warfighter serving. As a rule of thumb: one serving of fruit would be one apple, one banana, one orange, or one pear. One serving of grain products would be one slice of whole wheat bread or one bagel. In addition, one serving of vegetables would be ½ cup of peas, one small potato, or ½ cup of carrots. It is likely that Warfighters are eating more than one serving at each meal.

The second recommendation is more difficult, since it is difficult to know how much fiber is in each food, unless the amount is on a label, which does list the total amount of fiber.

When to Minimize Fiber Intake

Dietary fiber increases transit time, stool bulk and weight, and promotes regularity. During extended operations, "regular eliminations" may want to be **avoided** for as long as possible. A low-fiber diet may be preferred for these oc-

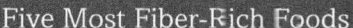

Five Most Fiber-Rich Foods

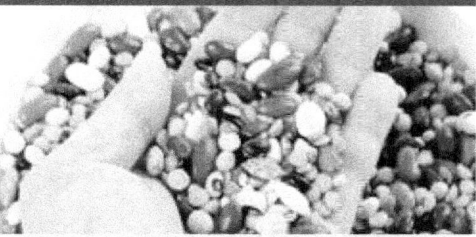

Legumes: 15–19 g/cup

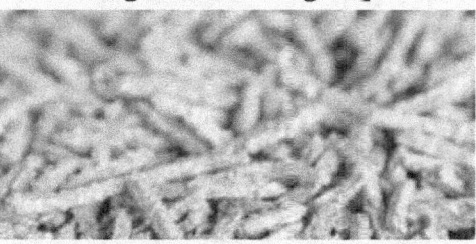

Wheat bran: 17 g/cup

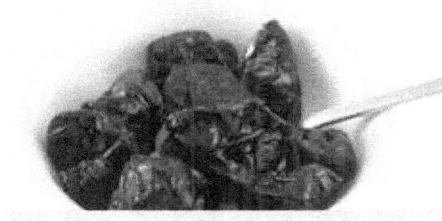

Prunes: 12 g/each

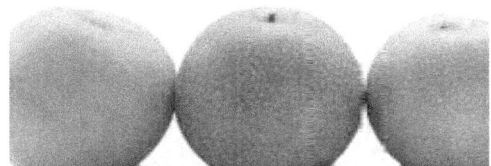

Asian pears: 10 g/pear

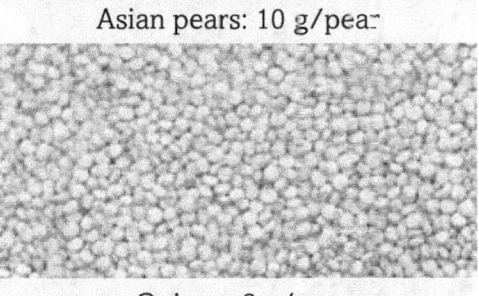

Quinoa: 9 g/cup

Eating more fruits and vegetables, whole wheat breads, whole grain cereals, beans, rice, nuts, and seeds is the best way to add fiber to your diet.

casions. Also, many high-fiber foods can cause bloating and gas if they are not regularly consumed, or if not enough water is consumed as well. High-fiber foods should be tested during training to find out how your system reacts. No dietary modifications should be tried before a mission or operational scenario.

Probiotics and Prebiotics

Probiotics and prebiotics are both of interest because they can help maintain a healthy gastrointestinal tract. Probiotics are live microorganisms (in most cases, bacteria) that help maintain the natural balance in the intestines and promote a healthy digestive system. Over 400 types of "good bacteria," "friendly bacteria," or intestinal flora reside in the human tract (lactic acid bacteria), where they reduce the effects of harmful bacteria.

Probiotics

Sources of Probiotics

Probiotics are found in real food, such as yogurt, kefir, and other cultured milk products, as well as added to capsules, tablets, beverages, and powders.

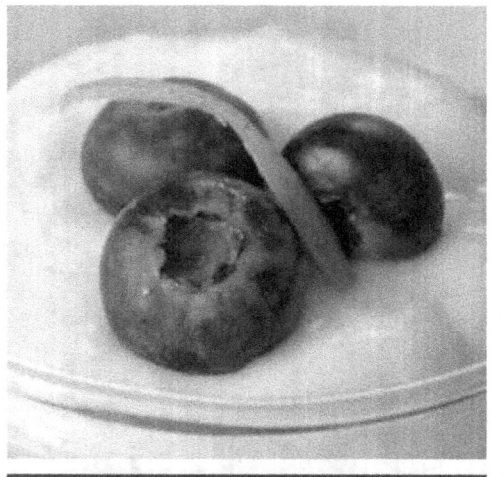

Yogurt: dairy product produced by bacterial fermentation of milk.	Fermented milk, such as buttermilk.
Unfermented milk.	Tempeh: fermented food made by the controlled fermentation of cooked soybeans with a Rhizopus mold.
Soy beverages.	Kefir: fermented milk drink.
Sauerkraut: finely sliced cabbage fermented by various lactic acid bacteria.	Kimchi: fermented dish made of seasoned vegetables, often cabbage.
Kombucha: sweetened tea or tisane that has been fermented by a macroscopic solid mass of microorganisms.	Miso: Japanese food produced by fermenting rice, barley and/ or soybeans, with salt and the mold.

Uses of Probiotics

Because "good bacteria" can be destroyed by antibiotics, illnesses, and other insults to the body, probiotics are sometimes used. For example, people use probiotics to prevent diarrhea caused by antibiotics. Although antibiotics eliminate harmful bacteria that may cause an illness, they also destroy the "good bacteria." A decrease in the number of beneficial bacte-

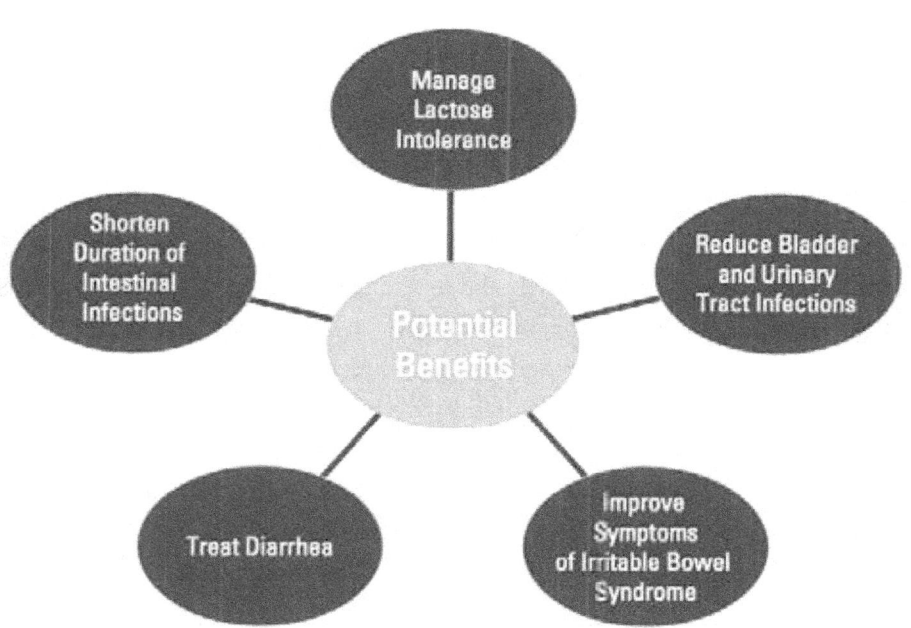

ria may lead to other complications, such as intestinal illnesses and flare-ups of inflammatory bowel disease. Taking probiotics may help replace the "good bacteria" that have been destroyed and restore the balance of "good" to "bad" bacteria. Some of the health claims of ingesting probiotics have been substantiated by research.

Purported health benefits of probiotics, when the probiotics are derived from food sources, include:

- Prevent colon cancer.

- Lower LDL "bad" cholesterol.

- Lower blood pressure.

- Improve immune function and prevent infections.

- Improve mineral absorption.

- Prevent harmful bacterial growth under stress.

Prebiotics

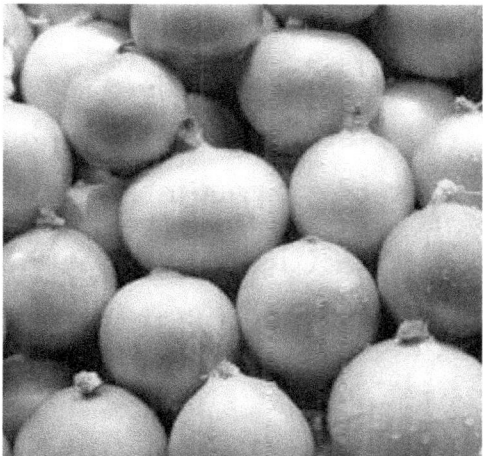

In contrast to probiotics, prebiotics are the fuels used by the bacteria present in the gastrointestinal tract. Prebiotics are non-digestible carbohydrates that selectively stimulate the growth and/or activity of beneficial bacteria (probiotics) in the colon. Unlike probiotics, prebiotics naturally occur in plants, such as garlic, asparagus, and onion. Other foods containing prebiotics include oatmeal, barley, beans, whole grains, leafy green vegetables, berries, yogurt, and milk. Two prebiotics added to many foods are inulin and fructo-oligosaccharides (FOS). Because prebiotics may boost the effects of probiotics, food manufactures have created synthetic prebiotics and added them to foods.

An Alkaline Diet

The energy-providing nutrients of all foods are carbohydrates, proteins, fats (and alcohol). They combine the four basic elements: carbon, nitrogen, hydrogen, and oxygen. When these nutrients are used for energy, they result in "acids," which need to be disposed of through urine, sweat, and the like. If too many acid-products are formed due to lifestyle behaviors and exposures (ingesting too much alcohol, overwork, over-indulgence, insufficient rest, inadequate water intake, tobacco use, pollution, etc.), the body has a difficult time removing all of them. Eating foods that are alkaline (such as fruits and vegetables that contain calcium, magnesium, sodium, potassium, etc.) can help remove excess acid. Overall, it is healthier to strive for a balanced middle ground—acid and alkaline foods. However, when under significant physical and mental stress, a diet high in alkaline foods is recommended.

The acidity of the body is usually determined by testing the first urine of the morning, before any food has been eaten. Urine tends to have wide variations (pH of 4.5–8) based on the acid or alkaline potential of foods eaten the day before. Blood is basically neutral or slightly alkaline (pH = 7.41). Urine strips can be purchased to test urine, but overall, it is best to select foods that are both acid and alkaline.

"The Warfighter is the primary weapons platform. There is an imperative to extend the operational life and maximize the battlefield performance of Warfighters. Nutrition is a critical component in human performance strategies."

CAPT "Pete" Van Hooser, Former Commodore, CNSWG-Two